GROUP THERAPY
FOR CANCER PATIENTS

GROUP THERAPY FOR CANCER PATIENTS

*A Research-Based Handbook
of Psychosocial Care*

DAVID SPIEGEL, M.D.

CATHERINE CLASSEN, PH.D.

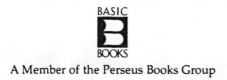

A Member of the Perseus Books Group

Published by Basic Books,
A Member of the Perseus Books Group

Library of Congress Cataloging-in-Publication Data
Spiegel, David, 1945-
   Group therapy for cancer patients / David Spiegel, Catherine Classen.
      p.   cm.
Includes bibliographical references and index.
ISBN 0-465-09565-8
   1. Cancer—Pyschological aspects.   2. Group psychotherapy.
3. Cancer—Patients—Mentalhealth.   I. Classen, Catherine, 1955-   II. Title.
RC271.P79 S67   1999
616.99'4'0019—dc21   99-049262

00 01 02 03 / 10 9 8 7 6 5 4 3

To Irv Yalom:
mentor, therapist, scholar and friend
—a man for all reasons.

Contents

PART III:
HELPING PATIENTS MANAGE
THEIR EXISTENTIAL CONCERNS

Acknowledgments

We are deeply grateful to the many patients with breast cancer and other illnesses and their families who have participated in our groups and without whom we would not have been able to write this book. Talented therapists have devoted themselves to our research program: Susan Diamond, L.C.S.W., A.C.S.W., Pat Fobair, L.C.S.W., Meg Marnell, Ph.D., Dhira Wallston, L.C.S.W., Susan Weisberg, L.C.S.W., and others. A dedicated staff has worked tirelessly to recruit and implement the studies: Casey AH, B.A.; Ami Atkinson, B.A.; Jane Benson, L.C.S.W.; Jennifer Boyce, B.A.; Karin Calde, B.A.; Vickie Chang, B.A.; Sanjay Chakrapani, B.A.; Julie Choe, B.A.; Diana Edwards, B.A.; Laurel Hill, M.A.; Hiroko Kameda, B.A.; Kris Kamikawa, B.A.; Trina Kurek, B.A.; Lynne LoPresto, M.A.; Elaine Miller, R.N., M.P.H.; Bita Nouriani, M.A.; Greg Schall, B.A.; Mike Schall, B.A.; Tukey Seagraves; Julie Seplaki, M.A.; Leslie Smithline, M.A.; Barbara Symons, B.A.; David Weibel, M.B.A.; Julia Zarcone, M.A.; and many others. An equally committed team of investigators has worked long hours to analyze the data from this and related projects: Karyn Angell, Ph.D.; Sophia Abramson, Ph.D.; Jane Blake-Mortiner, Ph.D.; Lisa Butler, Ph.D.; Sue DiMiceli, M.A.; Ron Duran, Ph.D.; Janine Giese-Davis, Ph.D.; Cheryl Gore-Felton, Ph.D.; Kaye Hermanson, Ph.D.; Pam Kato, Ph.D.; Manuela Kogan, M.D.; Cheryl Koopman, Ph.D.; Luciana Lagana, Ph.D.; Sandra Sephton, Ph.D.; Julie Turner-Cobb, Ph.D.; and Susan Wheeler, M.A.; along with many others. The following have provided expert consultation on our research: Helena Kraemer, Ph.D., professor of biostatistics in psychiatry; Daniel Stites, M.D., professor of laboratory medicine at the University of California, San Francisco; Gary Morrow, Ph.D., associate professor and director of the University of Rochester Cancer Center; Robert Carlson, M.D., professor of medicine/oncology at Stanford; Robert Sapolsky, Ph.D., professor of biology at Stanford; and Irvin Yalom, M.D., professor emeritus of psychiatry at Stanford. We are grateful to these individuals and to the many other staff, medical students, graduate students, undergraduates, and volunteers who have worked hard to help us unravel the process of helping cancer patients to cope better, and how this process is related to the progression of the disease.

This book was written in part during two sabbaticals (DS) with the gracious support of host institutions: The Institut Curie in Paris and the Bellagio Center of the Rockefeller Foundation in Italy. At Bellagio, Gianna Celli was gracious beyond measure. I am deeply grateful for the resources, intellectual atmosphere, critical ideas, and encouragement I received.

The term *supportive-expressive* was used before us by the eminent psychotherapy researcher, Dr. Lester Luborsky of the University of Pennsylvania. We are indebted to him both for his research and his willing consent to our use of the term. As he put it, this is a sign that we are occupying "common ground." Finally, we want to especially thank JoAnn Miller, Cindy Hyden, and Mary Dorian for their patience, commitment to the book, attention to detail, and editorial expertise.

GROUP THERAPY
FOR CANCER PATIENTS

Introduction

This book is more about living with cancer than dying of it. We have found in twenty years of working with the medically ill that facing fears rather than avoiding them reduces distress in the long run. Much of the work described here involves confronting the threat of death head-on, as an opportunity to reassess life, master fears, reorder priorities, revise relationships, and get the most out of the time that remains. There is no reason to expect cancer patients to be prepared to do this on their own.

The better we get at transforming terminal illnesses such as cancer and heart disease into chronic ones, the more people there will be who live with serious illness. Ultimately, however, the death rate will always be one per person; sooner or later, each of us will confront our own mortality and stand to benefit from the mobilization of social support and emotional comfort that can come from a well-structured support group.

In earlier times, life was shorter, the ravages of infectious disease were more widespread, and no institutions separated us from the sick and dying. Today, we hide death. We have constructed a world as far removed from threat as possible. We send terminally ill people to hospitals and sneak them out of their rooms in disguised gurneys when they die; many adults have little idea of what the dying process is like.

There is a kind of security in the mundane, which we nourish, yet somehow people who have been given a life-transforming diagnosis such as that of cancer are expected to know what to do. Imagine being taken away from the familiar and affirming worlds of family, friends, and work and becoming a stranger in a strange land, awaiting test results, reading stale magazines in waiting rooms, exposing your deepest concerns to relative strangers. Sleep is disrupted, energy declines, and fear replaces the customary shield of personal invulnerability. Factor in the threat to mortality, the possible loss of various bodily functions, choices among treatments that can nauseate, weaken, sterilize, mutilate (breast cancer patients specifically have to choose between breast-removal and intensive courses of radiation and chemotherapy, between a permanently altered body image and anxiety about recurrence or both). The treatment often feels far worse than the disease in the early stages of a serious illness and this can undermine confidence in medical intervention besides. Then there are the financial issues arising from loss of work and the cost of medical treatment, and also the anxiety, depression, pain, and confusion that make the other problems still harder to manage. Even our biomedical optimism views cure as the only worthy goal.

We have learned enough about the common problems affecting the medically ill that it makes sense to offer structured assistance. Is gathering in a group to discuss common fears an admission of defeat? Does it hamper hopefulness and undermine the positive attitude cultivated in "alternative" medicine literature? What good does it do to face the worst, rather than hope for the best?

Modern medicine is based on an acute disease/curative model. The ideal is our triumph over many bacterial infections through the introduction of effective antibiotics: diagnose, treat, and cure. Our very success in treating bacterial infections during the early part of the twentieth century provided a new model that radically changed medicine because it was overapplied, sabotaging the oldest adage, "To cure rarely, to relieve suffering often, to comfort always." Many illnesses remain incurable and have at best been transformed from terminal to chronic, yet physicians have rewritten their job descriptions: "To cure always, to relieve suffering if there is time, and to let someone else do the comforting."

While dramatic progress has been made in curing some cancers (Hodgkin's lymphoma, testicular cancer, childhood leukemias), and while it is reasonable in many other circumstances to be optimistic, people with cancer do have reason to worry, and relieving their suffering and providing comfort must resume their places as primary goals. This book is focused on *care*, whether cure is possible or not. The aim is to help patients learn from us and each other, to feel intensely supported at a time when illness makes them feel very much alone, to allow them to express and deal with feelings they may never have coped with before. The goal is to learn to face what is coming resolutely and creatively, to let the disease, its treatment, and the threat of death do the minimum necessary damage to their lives.

The school of thought that espouses a positive attitude (visualize little white blood cells eating cancer cells and they will be vanquished), and the theory that cancer fulfills some unexamined psychological tendency to self-destruction, speak to a common human need for a sense of control. That there is something people can do to direct the course of cancer in their bodies provides a certain kind of solace and the illusion of effective action. The desire for control is adaptive and can indeed be productively harnessed—by matching the efforts to the domains where action is demonstrably likely to be effective. We can control our levels of stress, our medical treatment decisions, our choices of friends, our perception of pain, but we cannot control the growth of tumors by visualizing their disappearance.

There is no evidence that such attitudes have anything to do with getting or dying of cancer. It is bad enough to get cancer without being blamed for it. We have great difficulty comprehending randomness. Trauma victims frequently retell the traumatic event in such a way that they become convinced they could have done something to avoid it, like the driver who says he should have turned left a block earlier instead of continuing down the road that led to the accident, or the rape victim who blames herself for not having foreseen the danger inflicted upon her by a predator. The core element in trauma is helplessness, the absolute inability to control what is happening.

We believe that facing fears in a supportive atmosphere can lead to overcoming them—that patients feel less alone and less helpless when they face their fears together; that the prepared patient is more able to manage life in the face of disease progression. That conviction is rooted in the findings of studies initiated in the 1970s, when Professor Irvin Yalom at Stanford decided to apply his considerable knowledge of group therapy to an existential problem: How do women with advanced breast cancer come to terms with their mortality? Could this period be life-enriching? Could facing death enhance life?

Recently, one of us (D.S.) presented this research to the Dalai Lama, and asked him why, from his spiritual perspective, women with advanced cancer seemed to do better when they faced each other's deaths directly and planned for their own. The Dalai Lama replied: "I have a very busy travel schedule and it makes me quite anxious. I wonder if I will be able to do all the things that are expected of me. When I am worried, I ask one of my assistants to explain to me what I will be doing for the next two days, and then I feel better, because I know what is ahead of me. That is the way we Buddhists feel about death. We spend much time preparing for it. In that way, it is no longer unfamiliar territory."

We can benefit from the tools we use to master other parts of life to tame our response to the prospect of dying. We can make it familiar territory, and do it in such a way that our fears and sadness are respected. We can feel more cared about and can gain ground on our fears. Indeed, such a confrontation with death can be a stimulus to a new kind of life, devoid of the everydayness with which we hide from existential dread (Yalom, 1980). In facing death directly, we can learn to trivialize the trivial, get rid of unwanted obligations, and focus on what matters: living life to the fullest while we can.

These lessons have been hard-earned. We and our colleagues have shared the sorrows and joys of many hundreds of cancer patients and their families over twenty years. They have given generously of their time, thoughts, and feelings to each other and to us, in the hope that what they have gone through will help others. In writing this book we are keeping a pact with them. Many have died; others live on and live well. They are indeed models of how openly and courageously you can live with cancer, facing the worst while hoping for the best.

In keeping with the premise that we live most authentically through an awareness of the fragility of our existence, Yalom maintained that confrontation with serious illness could be a period of growth rather than decline. We began our work with metastatic breast cancer patients to explore that premise, yet not without concern that face-to-face confrontation with the death of other group members from the same disease might seriously demoralize them. Such existential philosophers as Kierkegaard, Heidegger, Husserl, and Sartre held that it was only through a confrontation with the fragility of life that one truly lived, that existence was defined by nonexistence. You truly value living only when you can bring yourself to face the reality of dying.

Yalom brought together a research team that included Joan Bloom of the University of California at Berkeley, Regina Kriss, now a psychologist in private practice, Susan Weisberg, an oncology social worker at Stanford, and David Spiegel, the Stanford psychiatrist who is coauthor of this book. With initial support from the National Cancer Institute, a randomized trial of the effects of group psychotherapy was conducted. Eighty-six women with metastatic breast cancer were gathered, with considerable help from many oncologists, nurses, and social workers. All were tested at the beginning of the study, and thirty-six were randomly assigned to receive routine (and excellent) oncological care. The remaining fifty received this care plus a year of the weekly group psychotherapy described in the pages that follow.

We found that confronting even the worst allowed patients to examine their fears in a manner that proved helpful. They felt supported and understood, facing the ultimate isolation—death—together rather than alone. They came to see death as a series of problems rather than one big one. They worried more about the process of dying, which they could control, than about death itself, which they could not. They understood how they would be grieved as they mourned others in their group who died, and so saw death from the perspective of the bereaved as well as the dying.

The meetings were intense, often sad, at times amusing. We grieved together and came to care about each other quite deeply. We braced ourselves for losses, suffering through the deaths of group members, visiting in their homes as they lay near death, attending memorial services, dealing with the sinking feeling that comes with another loss. Yet the group itself survived for many years and it yielded a harvest of surprising results.

Despite being nose-to-nose with the deaths of group members with the same disease, our patients were less anxious and depressed, used less denial, and were less phobic at the end of the initial year than they were at the beginning, while the control patients receiving routine care had deteriorated emotionally (Spiegel, Bloom, et al., 1981). By the end of the initial year of the study, our group members also had half the pain of those in the control group on a self-rating scale they filled out periodically (two versus four out of a possible ten points; Spiegel and Bloom, 1983).

But the most striking and unexpected finding came ten years later, in the late 1980s, when we learned that the women randomly assigned to the treatment group had lived an average of eighteen months longer than the control patients after participating in the intervention (Spiegel, Bloom et al., 1989). Indeed, within four years after the study had begun, all of the control patients had died and a third of the treatment sample was still alive. Although eventually all but two of the patients died, it was clear that there was a difference in survival time, favoring the treatment group.

Did the group therapy cause prolonged survival time? Our Psychosocial Treatment Laboratory at Stanford is currently exploring this question with support from the National Institute of Mental Health, the National Cancer Institute, the John D. and Catherine T. MacArthur Foundation, the Fetzer Institute, the Nathan Cummings Foundation, and the Dana Foundation, among others. We have convened a new sample of 125 women with metastatic breast cancer who are participating in a similar randomized prospective trial. Although we are not yet ready to answer the survival question, we do have evidence that participating in these groups reduces psychological distress (Classen, Butler et al., in submission).

In a related multicenter trial supported by the National Cancer Institute and its Community Clinical Oncology Program, and in collaboration with Gary Morrow, Ph.D., of the University of Rochester Cancer Center, we are conducting a trial of a shorter version of this treatment—only twelve weeks—with 353 women who have been recently diagnosed with breast cancer at eleven sites across the United States. This study began in 1993 and is just being completed. We are finding that even this briefer form of group therapy benefits those women who are significantly distressed, and results in reduced anxiety and depression (Classen, Koopman et al., in submission). Our experience in this trial has helped us to refine and teach our method of supportive-expressive group therapy (Classen, Abramson et al., 1997). We have received wonderful cooperation and enthusiasm from the participating sites, and our data suggest that the method is teachable and learnable.

The bulk of our work has involved women with breast cancer, which is the paradigmatic problem we address in the book. However, there are many common medical, existential, and interpersonal issues for those with serious illness, and we believe that what we provide here is a template that can be applied to many other medical problems. Accordingly, we are exploring applications of this model to cancer of the prostate to see whether men could benefit as much as women from these groups. Reasoning that many of the psychosocial problems—isolation, fear, the need to redefine life goals—are quite similar for all these patient groups, we have applied this group approach to individuals with cardiac arrhythmias, multiple sclerosis, bone marrow transplants, and also, under the direction of Cheryl Koopman, Ph.D., HIV infection. Selected additional studies are cited at the end of the introduction.

The supportive-expressive model has also been examined in other laboratories:

1. The BEST (Breast Expressive-Supportive Trial), a Canadian Multicenter Group Therapy Trial for Metastatic Breast Cancer Patients, is directed by Pamela Goodwin, M.D. (Goodwin, Leszcz et al., 1996). Funded by the Medical Research Council of Canada, this trial involves 225 women at seven sites across Canada and is intended as a

replication trial of our initial findings that breast cancer patients given group therapy had longer survival. The group psychotherapy is supervised by Dr. Molyn Leszcz.

2. Supportive/Expressive and Cognitive/Behavioral Group Therapy for Breast Cancer Patients is a study being conducted by David Kissane, M.D., and funded by the Australian Cancer Board. It is a comparison of supportive-expressive and cognitive-behavioral group therapies at Monash University in Melbourne to evaluate psychological and medical effects of group therapy for women with primary breast cancer.

3. A trial of group therapy and antidepressant (SSRI) treatment for metastatic breast cancer patients is being conducted by Anders Bonde, M.D., and Per Beck, M.D., in Denmark. This study is designed to compare effects of antidepressants and group therapy in 200 metastatic breast cancer patients.

4. Marc Archinard, M.D., is conducting a replication trial of our original study in Geneva, funded by the Swiss Cancer League.

5. A randomized multisite trial in Canada examining the benefits of supportive-expressive group therapy for lupus patients is being conducted by Patricia Dobkin, Ph.D.

6. David Mohr, Ph.D., is conducting an intervention trial for multiple sclerosis patients with major depressive disorder at the University of California, San Francisco, funded by the National Multiple Sclerosis Society. His patients are randomly assigned to three treatment groups: supportive-expressive group therapy, individual cognitive-behavioral therapy, or treatment with sertraline (Zoloft).

7. A randomized trial comparing supportive-expressive group therapy, anthroposophic treatment and standard care is being conducted by Thomas Cerny, M.D. and colleagues in Bern, Switzerland. This trial is examining the effect of complementary therapies on quality of life and survival.

This book shares treatment techniques designed to make the most of group psychotherapeutic intervention for the medically ill. It is primarily for those who run these groups or plan to in the future. We hope that health professionals from medicine, nursing, psychology, social work, and other allied disciplines will find it useful. We also hope that it will be of help to the burgeoning self-help and group support movement, although the groups in the book are designed to be leader-led. We assume some familiarity with the general principles of psychotherapy: the relationship as a therapeutic tool; the idea of transference; distortions of perception in relationships; the Sullivanian concept that a psychotherapist is both a participant in a patient's life, with real feelings and concerns, and an observer as well. We also assume some medical knowledge regarding the range of medical treatments. We assume a fundamental respect for the primacy of the doctor-patient relationship—our group treatments are designed to facilitate medical care. We recognize that any given reader may be more thoroughly trained in one of these areas than another, and for this reason we encourage group co-leadership so that the range of knowledge from psychotherapy to oncology is better covered.

Chapter 1 addresses the distress and depression that accompanies a diagnosis of cancer, and the importance of social support is emphasized. The justification for support groups is highlighted in Chapter 2 by case examples.

The therapist is provided with guidelines for group leadership in Chapter 3 and with treatment strategies in Chapter 4. Chapter 5 suggests ways to facilitate supportive interactions among group members and how to handle problematic expressions of support among members. One of the key features of the therapist's work in support groups is encouraging the open expression of emotion among members, which is covered in Chapter 6 with examples.

In Chapter 7 we cover issues related to discussions of death and dying. Chapter 8 is focused on helping patients with the profound feelings of isolation that arise from having a life-threatening illness. We describe existential concerns related to freedom, such as "How shall I redefine myself now that I have cancer?" Assisting patients in the struggle to make meaning out of their transformed lives is the focus of Chapters 7 and 8.

Suggestions for facilitating family and specialized groups are provided in Chapter 9. Common group problems are explored in Chapter 10—for example, how to handle a group member's decision to discontinue therapy and how to deal with confrontations between group members. Finally, hypnosis techniques for pain control are outlined in Chapter 11.

When we started this research in the 1970s, our biggest problem was convincing cancer patients to donate an hour and a half a week to joining a group. The control patients were quite content to undergo routine care. Today, happily, we have the opposite problem. Most patients do not want to be assigned to the control group—they want group therapy. Many self-help and mutual support groups are springing up around the country, urged on by organizations such as Y-Me, the National Coalition of Cancer Survivorship, the Cancer Support Community in San Francisco, the Wellness Community, and many other extremely helpful patient organizations. More and more oncology programs are including groups as part of their treatment. It is our hope that this text will facilitate the application and availability of this kind of support for many women and men with cancer and other life-threatening diseases. We want to see the day come when group support is not an add-on or an afterthought, but a routine part of medical care. Whether such support helps cancer patients live longer, it is by now indisputable that it helps them live better. We hope that our experience will enrich yours.

One of us (D.S.) spent a sabbatical at the Institut Curie in Paris working with the genetic research team of Gilles Thomas, Ph.D., and Dominique Stoppa-Lyonnet, Ph.D. This team is defining portions of the recently discovered BrCA1 gene correlated with genetic risk for the disease in an effort to better understand the phenomenology and mechanisms of the heritability of this breast and ovarian cancer risk. We developed a group model for women recently diagnosed with breast cancer who are also at familial risk (Classen, Diamond et al., 1994), and therefore have special problems involving having lost family members to the same disease, and the pervasive concerns about passing the risk on to their children.

We also had the opportunity to test the supportive/expressive model in a different culture and language. Co-led by Sylvie Schwab, Ph.D., the groups were well received.

PART ONE
RATIONALE FOR
INVOLVING CANCER PATIENTS
IN GROUP SUPPORT

CHAPTER 1

Experiencing Cancer

In this chapter we discuss the plight of the cancer patient, documenting the emotional, informational, and social needs elicited by the illness, and the need for a group support program to address these issues.

We are fundamentally social creatures. We derive much of our sense of well-being, importance, and value through the daily response of others to us. It is rare for humans to live alone, or even to spend much time alone. Yet somehow, especially in Western culture, we define ourselves primarily as individuals who make occasional forays into the social world. How thoroughly dependent we are on our social networks becomes clear when we are separated from them. A diagnosis of cancer or other life-threatening illness disrupts social contact in many ways. It removes people from customary contacts because of time away from work, school, and family. Cancer patients are suddenly entering a new and strange social system. Furthermore, the isolation is bidirectional. Many acquaintances, friends, and even family are awkward about illness, not knowing what to say, fearful for the ill person and for themselves. The cancer patient has to learn a new set of social roles, just as comfortable old ones are pulled away.

As a society we recognize that most new roles in life require some training: driving a car, accepting a new job, joining a religious congregation. We have little or no formal preparation for becoming a cancer patient, however, leading to considerably more distress than is necessary. Certainly the illness itself is understandably stressful, carrying with it the threat of death, the need for uncomfortable and possibly disfiguring treatments, and the disruption of everyday life. However, the loss of social support at such a time can reinforce the other stressors, leaving cancer patients suddenly ill and feeling very much alone with their concerns.

We are often sequestered from dying and death in the modern world. Many have never seen a dead body, few have attended to loved ones during their terminal illness, and death in our culture is viewed as an aberration rather than a natural part of life—something to be ashamed of rather than faced directly. Thus, the diagnosis of cancer usually catches us not merely frightened but unprepared. It is never easy to cope with cancer, but it can be done effectively and well. Relatively less attention has been paid to this human side of living with the disease, the person and body fighting the cancer. Medicine has focused more on attacking the disease itself. Here we chart a course of support for cancer patients involving group psychotherapy. We begin with an examination of the experience of having cancer.

THE DIAGNOSIS

A thirty-five-year-old secretary consulted a surgeon after a mammogram that showed a 3 millimeter lesion in her right breast. He confirmed the presence of the tumor by palpation and review of the mammogram, and recommended an open biopsy. She began to shake and cry. "We don't have to do the biopsy if it upsets you," he said. He was attempting to calm her down. But what he was really doing was forcing her panic inward. He held her arm and tried to reassure her: "Most of these lumps are benign. Don't worry now." Of course, she was worried. The very magnitude of her fear seemed to her a measure of the danger. Such strong emotion is information as well as expression, a confirmation of how serious the problem is. And all too often in medicine, even the most caring physicians confuse inducing external calm with putting fears to rest.

A surgeon who would never simply cover up an infected wound will instinctively suppress the anguish that is naturally associated with a diagnosis of cancer. This leaves newly diagnosed (and other) cancer patients to fend for themselves emotionally. It also gives them the impression that such feelings are inappropriate, a sign of their personal deficiency in coping, rather than a natural reaction to an acute threat to bodily integrity, family, work, and recreation—indeed, to life itself.

The doctor might have helped his patient more had he said to her: "I know this is upsetting. We don't yet know whether the lump is malignant or not. But whatever it is, I will help you take care of it." This response would acknowledge and accept her distress, assure her of ongoing support no matter what happened, and indicate that no matter what the result of the biopsy, there was a great deal that could be done to address the problem.

Cancer induces a special kind of fear—that of the body turning on itself, of normal cells becoming enemies and attacking others. It is a disease fraught with uncertainty and helplessness. For many it can feel like a death sentence. Along with the sheer dread that cancer may kill, there are many other ramifications. These include dealing with medical treatment of the disease, coping with a changed self-image, and managing the impact of the illness on family, friends, and work relationships.

The very intensity of the feelings elicited by the diagnosis of cancer sets in motion strong forces, both intrapsychic and interpersonal, against the expression of these feelings. Many patients feel as though controlling their emotions about cancer is a means of controlling the disease itself: "It can't be too serious if I don't let it upset me." "If I let the illness get me down, it will progress more rapidly." Some patients have incorporated the popular notion that a consistently positive attitude can cure their cancer. One patient told her psychotherapy group that her husband said, "Don't cry—you'll make the cancer spread." The group subsequently referred to his comment as "the prison of positive thinking."

Nonetheless, negative feelings associated with cancer are almost as unwelcome as the illness itself. They may become a symbolic battleground for the degree to which the cancer encroaches on life. At first, many cancer patients struggle with an all-or-none view of its emotional effects. The diagnosis is so devastating that the possibility of ever having any pleasure again seems remote at best. Many try to remain strong and in control so as not to be overwhelmed with fear and anxiety. The only way to maintain some homeostasis seems to be to try to put the threat aside and act as though nothing has happened. However, fear, sadness, anxiety, and other disease-related emotions creep in, intruding on awareness in the same way that memories of a traumatic stressor do on crime and accident victims.

The need to retain a strong and composed attitude comes from outside pressures as well. Partners and family members may unintentionally communicate the wish that the patient be strong because otherwise emotion in the patient may elicit similar uncomfortable feelings in family members. When the patient is strong this helps the family members to cope with their own feelings of helplessness and fear. This dynamic tends to reinforce the isolation both patients and their family members feel in dealing with the threat of cancer.

Indeed, the same struggle for emotional control often affects partners, parents, and children. They frequently feel the need to be strong as well so as not to upset their loved one who is ill. For a husband or child to cry would be an admission of how serious the threat is. But it is also an admission of love and concern. Admitting that you are afraid does not mean that the worst will happen. However, to avoid sharing such concerns means that at a crucial time—during disease diagnosis or progression, for example—family members may suffer in silence, each alone with their anxiety, rather than comforting each other together.

Sometimes symptoms of distress are hidden rather than obvious. This can mislead physicians and family to the mistaken belief that everything is fine, that the patient is taking the diagnosis very well. The cancer patient's reaction to the news can be composed of denial and disbelief. Upon being told that she had breast cancer, one woman went into such a deep state of denial that she "forgot" about it and "remembered" six months later, finally seeking treatment. Although such extensive denial is unusual, other forms of denial are not. A more common form is believing there must be some mistake, that the patient has been confused with someone else. Such initial responses may buffer the individual from the fear that reality imposes temporarily, but they may also interfere with obtaining necessary treatment and support.

Like any traumatic event, the response to a cancer diagnosis can include a variety of dissociative, intrusive, avoidance, and hyperarousal symptoms, often seen in individuals with an acute or posttraumatic stress disorder (American Psychiatric Association, 1994). These include a class of numbing and avoidance symptoms, in which the individual seems to avoid exposing herself or himself to, or reacting to, stimuli that are reminders of the traumatic information. Such apparent underreaction can have two important consequences. First, it can lead family, friends, and health care professionals to underestimate the magnitude of the impact of the illness on the patient. Second, a lack of appropriate emotional response to a stressor can lead to more severe symptomatology. For example, studies of combat stress response and victims of a firestorm have both indicated that numbing, the lack of emotional response to the trauma, is a strong predictor of the development of later posttraumatic stress disorder (PTSD) (Koopman, Classen et al., 1994; McFarlane, 1986; Bremner, Southwick et al., 1992; Marmar, Weiss et al., 1994; Solomon and Mikulincer, 1988; Lindemann, 1944 [94]).

Recent research has documented the intrusion and avoidance symptoms of PTSD among patients with cancer (Butler, Koopman et al., in press; DuHamel, Redd et al., 1996; Krupnick, 1996). Indeed, among some patients with histories of earlier traumatic stressors, diagnosis and treatment of medical illness can initiate a recrudescence of symptoms of PTSD (Baider, Peretz et al., 1992; Spiegel and Kato, 1996; Spiegel and Classen, 1995). Thus, putting the distressing information out of sight does not put it out of mind, and it makes the cancer patient more vulnerable to later intrusive avoidance and hyperarousal symptoms.

The emotional dynamics evoked by the illness can also contaminate the doctor–patient interaction. Consider the implications of a cancer diagnosis from a simple behavioral/classical-conditioning perspective. A patient goes to a physician with what is presented as a minor complaint—a lump, for example, or some bleeding. Suddenly, it is transformed into a life threat through the physician's tests, touch, and words. The patient is strongly negatively reinforced for bringing up the complaint; if the doctor also rejects the patient's natural emotional response, the negative reinforcement is doubled. Without even knowing it, the patient will be less inclined in the future to bring further symptoms, no matter how innocent or important, to the physician's attention. Experience can be a grim teacher: If the "punishment" is not worked through, the sense of threat can become an obstacle to future collaboration with physicians and others on the health care team. Addressing emotional concerns early and often is a good way preempt damage to the doctor–patient relationship.

A CHANGED SELF-IMAGE

The diagnosis of cancer along with its treatment has a profound effect on a person's self-image. Despite doctors' efforts to buffer the effect of the diagnosis—"Cancer is a word, not a sentence"—it has profound implications. The shock of the diagnosis, the whirlwind of treatment, and the adjustment to a radically altered body as a result of surgery, radiotherapy, chemotherapy, and hormonal treatment leave the patient little opportunity to integrate the changes into his or her conception of self.

Prior to the diagnosis, many patients are in relatively good health. As one breast surgeon put it, being told you have cancer is "like being shot by a sniper." Thus, the new role of cancer patient must be assimilated, together with the loss of a sense of invulnerability. This can present a significant challenge to self-esteem as it typically raises issues of dependency, inadequacy, and frailty.

Cancer and its treatment leave patients with limited energy and compromised physical abilities. For those used to feeling independent and self-sufficient, being in the position of requiring help with what were once minor tasks can be upsetting. For those who are athletic, viewing themselves as physically fit and full of energy no longer matches their present capabilities. An important goal for cancer patients should be to adjust their internalized vision of themselves so that it more accurately mirrors their actual abilities. Part of the distress is the gap between expectation and reality.

While some changes, such as the experience of constant fatigue, are temporary, the drive to feel "normal" and act as though nothing serious has happened can push cancer patients to expect more of themselves than is realistic, or to be unduly self-critical if they cannot carry on a normal life on top of medical illness and treatment. Changes such as losing hair during chemotherapy or having a mastectomy can leave the patient with the sense of her body as unfamiliar, damaged, and even menacing; in the breast cancer patient, they can have a powerful effect on a woman's sense of her own femininity and attractiveness. Accepting her new body and integrating it into a healthy and positive self-image are important.

Identifying and grieving for what has been irrevocably altered or lost is a necessary part of coming to terms with the change wrought by cancer. These losses need to be grieved for, in part by working through how they have altered the cancer patients' sense of themselves (Spiegel, 1979). They must grieve for the life they once had, recognizing that things can never be quite the same. However, as priorities are readjusted, patients can find that life also becomes better in many ways.

STRESS AND DISTRESS

Cancer can be understood as, among other things, a series of stressors: the diagnosis, arduous treatments, fear of death, changes in social and physical environment. Each of these stressors alone is taxing enough. For the cancer patient, however, the seemingly endless barrage of stressors affects all aspects of life, beginning with what at first can seem like a death sentence. There is the stress of needing to make urgent and crucial decisions that have the potential to affect one's very survival. Oftentimes there is disfiguring surgery and then the pain and discomfort of chemotherapy and radiation, and such side effects as hair loss or lymphedema and a fatigue that has never before been experienced. There is the disruption to work and home environment. There may be problems with health insurance. There may be concerns about the effect of the illness on family members and the cancer patient's simultaneous needs to protect them and depend on their support. Most cancer patients undergo at least transient serious distress; a substantial proportion continue to experience significant anxiety and depression.

THE LITERATURE ON DISTRESS

While several early studies showed good long-term adjustment of breast cancer patients (Craig and Abeloff, 1974; Schottenfeld and Robbins, 1970), others demonstrated that 20 to 30 percent of patients suffer severe distress for two years or more postsurgery (Ganz, Lee et al., 1992; Browne et al., 1990). For example, as many as 80 percent of breast cancer patients report significant distress during initial treatment (Hughes, 1982). Even years later, 10 percent continue to have severe maladjustment (Omne-Ponten, Holmberg et al., 1992). Surprisingly, in breast cancer patients, breast-sparing surgery does not reduce the rate of emotional disturbance (Fallowfield, Baum et al., 1987; Levy, Herberman et al., 1989; Omne-Ponten, Holmberg et al., 1994). Elevated rates of mood disturbance have been observed throughout the course of the disease, from the time of undiagnosed breast lumps (Greer and Morris, 1975; Morris and Greer, 1982; Hughes, Royle et al., 1986) to recurrence (Hughes, Royle et al., 1986; Holland and Holland, 1989). Particular points of stress include recency of diagnosis and more advanced disease (Vinokur, Threatt et al., 1989).

THE LITERATURE ON PSYCHIATRIC DISORDERS

As many as 50 percent of cancer patients experience distress severe enough to warrant a psychiatric diagnosis, most commonly of depression and anxiety (Morris, Greer et al., 1977). The rate of depression is up to four times higher among oncology patients than in the general population (Mermelstein and Lesko, 1992). Furthermore, some 10 percent of patients suffer severe maladjustment to diagnosis and treatment and remain symptomatic six years later (Omne-Ponten, Holmberg et al., 1994).

In a study of 215 randomly selected oncology inpatients from three cancer centers, Derogatis and colleagues (Derogatis, Morrow et al., 1983) assessed the prevalence of psychiatric disorders. Of these patients, 47 percent were assessed to have psychiatric disorders; of those, 6 percent had major affective disorders and the remainder had adjustment disorders with depressed mood or mixed emotional features. Almost 90 percent of these psychiatric disorders were judged to be manifestations of or reactions to the disease or its treatment.

In another large study, breast cancer patients at one-year follow-up were compared with women who had undergone cholecystectomy, a breast biopsy with benign outcome, and healthy women (Study, 1987). Significantly higher somatic distress, self-denigration, psychosocial impairment, and physical complaints in the breast cancer patients were found, although the rate of psychiatric illness was not higher in those women who had good prior mental health. In a community study of 274 breast cancer patients, Vinokur and colleagues (Vinokur, Threatt et al., 1990) found that mental health problems including anxiety, depression, and somatic preoccupation persisted throughout the year after diagnosis. Interestingly, appraisal of threat was found to be a stronger predictor of mental health than initial stage of disease. The authors concluded that better education of patients might have the potential to reduce long-term distress.

THE LITERATURE ON DEPRESSION

Factors associated with increased levels of depression include degree of physical disability, presence of pain, and severity of illness. As disease progresses, the percentage of patients who are clinically depressed increases. For example, among the chronically medically ill, the rate of major depression is twice as high as the population base rate of 3 to 4 percent among medical outpatients, and reaches 12 percent among medical inpatients (Katon and Sullivan, 1990). Twenty percent of terminally ill patients are depressed, and the number rises to 60 percent among those requesting physician-assisted suicide (Chochinov, Wilson et al., 1995).

In random samples of hospitalized cancer patients, rates of depressive states have been found between 16 percent and 50 percent (Derogatis, Morrow et al., 1983; Greer, 1991; Lansky, List et al., 1985; Massie and Holland, 1987). In general, the more narrowly the term *depression* is defined, the less depression is reported. Mermelstein and colleagues (Mermelstein and Lesko, 1992) found that the rate of depression in their sample of cancer patients was as high as four times that of the general population.

The Literature on Anxiety

The rate of clinically significant anxiety disorders among cancer patients has been found to be as high as 14 percent (Maraste, Brandt et al., 1992). The most common specific problems are anxiety about recurrence (Koocher and O'Malley, 1981; Mahon, Cella et al., 1990; Quigley, 1989; Rieker, Edbril et al., 1985), sexual problems (Fallowfield and Hall, 1991; Maguire, Lee et al., 1978; Morris, Greer et al., 1977), death anxiety (Spiegel and Glafkides, 1983), and work-related difficulties (Fobair, Hoppe et al., 1986; Tross and Holland, 1990). The treatment itself also triggers recurrent anxiety, which may exacerbate conditioned anticipatory nausea (Cella, Pratt et al., 1986) and reduce adherence to medical treatment (Itano, Tanabe et al., 1983a, 1983b).

Obstacles to Effective
Diagnosis and Treatment

Why are emotional problems often overlooked and undertreated? There is an important problem in assessing psychiatric disturbance among the medically ill: Many of the symptoms of depression or anxiety appear to be by-products of the illness. Hopelessness can be considered a reaction to bad medical prognosis, fatigue to a side effect of radiotherapy, loss of appetite to chemotherapy, anhedonia to altered life circumstances. Thus, both the neurovegetative signs (weight loss, sleep disturbance) and emotional/cognitive signs of depression are often attributed to the medical illness itself (Craig, Comstock et al., 1974).

To some extent, complications of medical treatment do produce those symptoms. But they do not mitigate the presence of diagnosable and treatable mental disorders. While in theory such problems could lead to an excess of psychiatric diagnosis, in practice they more often allow physicians and others to discount real depressive and anxiety symptoms, thereby losing opportunities for effective treatment. In fact, depression in patients with cancer has been underdiagnosed and undertreated in part because of the belief that depression is a normal and universal reaction to serious disease

(Rodin and Voshart, 1986). The use of testing for biological markers of depression is a promising means of detecting and more effectively treating depression among cancer patients (McDaniel, Musselman et al., 1995).

EFFECTS OF EMOTIONAL DISTURBANCE ON MEDICAL TREATMENT

Cognitive deficits such as pseudodementia and impaired concentration are, like hopelessness and diminished energy, common in depression, and together they reduce adherence to treatment regimens. Efficacious treatments for disease-related anxiety and depression should reduce not only their prevalence and severity but also the symptoms that impair patients' ability to comprehend and adhere to effective oncological treatment.

Such patients, called *distressed high utilizers*, may place substantially extra demands on treating physicians, despite (or because of) their suboptimal use of medical information (Von Korff, Ormel et al., 1992). Poor adjustment to illness can increase the cost of medical care as much as 75 percent (Browne et al., 1990). Developing programmatic interventions to provide psychosocial support with appropriate psychotherapeutic and psychopharmacologic treatment would make the delivery of medical care more efficient while reducing patient discomfort and improving coping ability.

SOCIAL ISOLATION

Francine was attending an elegant garden party at the home of a friend in Atherton, California. She had been diagnosed with breast cancer some years earlier and had suffered a recurrence. Despite a course of chemotherapy and radiation therapy, she had felt well enough to attend the large gathering. In the middle of an otherwise pleasant afternoon, she looked down and noticed that her hostess had handed her a drink in a plastic cup, while everyone else was drinking out of a glass. Apparently, her hostess had been afraid of catching breast cancer were she to drink out of the same glass. Suddenly, Francine felt very much alone, like a source of fear and contamination rather than a friend.

A complaint often heard from cancer patients is that they feel isolated. They often feel they have moved from the mainstream into a world teeming with confusion and uncertainty. There is a sudden sense of being separated from the people to whom they were closest, of being catapulted from a relatively normal and healthy environment shared comfortably with loved ones into a world of disease and an uncertain future.

Many patients feel that few understand the crisis they are experiencing, that suddenly a chasm has opened between them and everyone who has the privilege of immersing themselves in the mundane. Everyday concerns are suddenly trivial. It seems a luxury to be able to worry about such things. Relating to other people can be difficult because their experience seems so different; indeed it is so different. And other people, in turn, seem to treat the person with cancer differently.

The isolation is bidirectional. Both cancer and death are on everyone's mind, but no one discusses them for fear of inducing an emotional reaction, of causing pain instead of uncovering and helping with it. Even well-meaning family and friends do not know what to say. Moreover, the occurrence of cancer in another necessarily arouses unpleasant emotions in the "unaffected" individual. Many friends feel an uneasy sense of victory over the person who is ill; inwardly relieved that the shoe has dropped elsewhere, and they also feel guilty.

Thus after a diagnosis of cancer, most relationships change. They either get better—more intense and caring—or they get worse, but they rarely stay the same. Old rituals suddenly seem hollow and meaningless; maintaining a semblance of normalcy when everything is different does not work well at all. Adjusting to the new realities is often a difficult and emotionally taxing process for family and friends.

SOCIAL SUPPORT

Serious medical illness is a test of any support network. Initially there is considerable stress over the problem of whom to tell; clearly, more intimate family and friends learn first about serious illness. The information is shared to cultivate instrumental and emotional support because it is crucial to those suddenly afflicted to feel cared about—to know that others are worried about them and stand ready to help.

Studies of sources of social support for cancer patients indicate that most women confide in women friends or relatives and in partners (Faller, Schilling et al., 1995) and rarely seek out mental health care settings for disclosure of their concerns. Interestingly, most women report feeling understood best by women friends rather than by partners. Their greater comfort in expressing their concerns to women may be related to body image changes following the removal of a breast, or may reflect findings that women are superior sources of emotion-focused social support.

Men suffer surprisingly similar problems in relation to cancer and social support. However, the barriers to direct expression of distress among men are even higher than those found among women. In a study of 327 prostate cancer patients, da Silva (1993) found that their sense of overall well-being was most affected by a reduced social life, impaired sexual potency, and fatigue. The interaction between sexual and social life on the one hand and distress on the other is clear (Borghede and Sullivan, 1996; DeAntoni and Crawford, 1994). While some have wondered whether men would respond to group interventions as well as women do, there is growing evidence that they need, will accept, and can benefit from group support (Sharp, Blum et al., 1993).

The type of social support available to cancer patients varies with the stage of the disease's progress (Dakof and Taylor, 1990). Early in the course of the disease, the need may be greatest for informational support, which is often not available in the cancer patient's social network. As they go through medical treatment, cancer patients may turn to family and friends for instrumental support to get to doctors' appointments, look after children, and manage the household while also requiring emotional support.

Despite the apparent support available to cancer patients through formal and informal means, the demands of the illness and treatment regimen often decrease opportunities for broad support networks (Bloom and Spiegel, 1984). Cancer-related pain, for example, leads to decreased physical and social activity. Although patients often report feeling supported by friends and family, 85 percent of cancer patients in one sample reported less self-initiated contact with friends and 65 percent reported that they isolated themselves due to the intensity of their pain (Strang and Qvarner, 1990). Such impediments to family communication are of particular concern since research suggests that social support can have protective effects on physical health (Berkman, Leo-Summers et al., 1992).

The kinds of psychiatric problems already noted, including depression and anxiety, may impair the amount of support obtained from families, which can, in turn, deepen these symptoms (Bloom, 1982). Several studies have shown the adverse impact of patient depression on family communication (Lewis and Hammond, 1992). For families in which a patient remains depressed, the marital relationship and family functioning suffer (Lewis and Hammond, 1992). In some cases, even increased family communication does not help the patient: For some cancer patients, increased communication with supportive others regarding the cancer was actually related to *lower* self-esteem (Faller, Schilling et al., 1995). While this is not a causal relationship (i.e., communication cannot be said to have caused lowered self-esteem), something may be missing in these usually supportive relationships.

However, a second study showed that sensitizing the supportive others to the emotional and physical needs of the cancer patient eliminated the relationship between better communication and poorer self-esteem in the patient. This raises three points. First, not all social relationships are supportive, nor are all supportive relationships consistent in the level of support they provide to the medically ill. Second, family and other relationships may change after a member is diagnosed with cancer. Many patients report feeling isolated within previously close relationships due to the new existential issues and needs facing them. Third, interventions within the family and other support systems can produce larger positive effects on the quality of support received. In other words, it may not be enough for someone who is ill to communicate their needs and problems. It is equally important that the family be helped to understand those problems and to figure out ways of addressing them.

The disease may force changes in the availability of social networks (Wortman and Dunkel-Schetter, 1979). Friends and family are often upset, ambivalent, frightened, and confused by the intrusion of cancer. Not uncommonly, they may avoid the issue of cancer or even withdraw from the patient altogether (Wortman and Dunkel-Schetter, 1979). Especially in these circumstances, more stable relationships (e.g., spouses and physicians) are usually resistant to the destabilizing effects of the illness, whereas other support sources—such as more distant relatives, friends, and acquaintances—may more easily slip away (Dakof and Taylor, 1990). This makes the disruption of long-term relationships with physicians under managed care, HMOs, and other forms of business reorganization of medicine all the more damaging (Richmond, Berman et al., 1996; Pelletier, Marie et al., 1997; Spiegel, Stroud et al., 1998). The rule with medical illness is that good relationships improve whereas bad or superficial ones often get worse. Losing contact with a trusted physician at a time of major illness seriously undermines support at a time when it is needed most.

Although social support for the medically ill is important to their quality of life, it may recede or not accommodate to the changes dictated by serious illness. Many people with cancer and other life-threatening illnesses feel alone in a crowd. Even those fortunate enough to be surrounded by loved ones may not get the help they need. Group support entails a means of both providing additional social support and modeling better means of obtaining good support from other existing social networks.

CONCLUSION

Cancer stirs a whirlpool of emotional and social problems. It stimulates emotional dysregulation and triggers a variety of efforts to manage strong feelings, some of which only perpetuate such feelings and hamper coping abilities. It intensifies the need for emotional, instrumental, and informational support at a time when support networks may be changing, as family and friends struggle to come to terms with the meaning of the illness.

The realities of the illness and its treatment are only one part of the life of someone with cancer or another life-threatening illness. Patients are challenged to manage their emotional reaction to this new state of disease, reorganize their life priorities, get through treatment, redefine their social support network, help their loved ones deal with their illness, and obtain new kinds of social support given their new needs. These problems cannot be handled with a simple prescription, and form the basis of a rationale for group intervention.

CHAPTER 2

Goals and Effects of Group Support

The use of support groups in the facilitation of coping with physical illness is relatively new. In the past, the emphasis has been on improving the doctor–patient relationship and providing individual counseling and psychotherapy for patients with the most serious emotional problems. Patients in need of help in adjusting to their illnesses sought consultation from their physicians, or received individual assistance from nurses, social workers, clergy, psychologists, or psychiatrists; much valuable support has been provided in this manner. Emphasis, however, continued to be on occasional individual consultation, privacy, and confidentiality. Supportive and psychotherapeutic interventions were the exception, not the rule. Furthermore, whatever contact one cancer patient had with another was incidental: in waiting rooms, shared hospital rooms, or through having a friend or family member with a similar illness.

There is no doubt that for some cancer patients individual counseling or psychotherapy remains the preferred avenue of assistance out of a desire for privacy, because of unusual or extreme problems, or because of the severity of psychiatric symptoms. Many others, however, are finding strength in numbers. They discover that they can use their experience with cancer to give as well as receive support. They find it invigorating to care about others in a similar situation, and to feel cared about in turn. They learn that their particular fears, discomforts, and experiences of rejection are common to the life of the cancer patient, thereby "normalizing" their reactions. They choose from an array of alternative coping strategies presented to them, and they construct a new network of social support. While some of these benefits may come naturally in the social environment, or in individual counseling or psychotherapy, they are the stock in trade of support groups, which is one likely reason that they are proliferating at a rapid rate.

Before cancer patients can begin to integrate their changed sense of who they are as people and of themselves physically, they must get over the initial shock and horror at what has unfolded for them. For women with breast cancer, sharing these experiences and hearing the stories of other women with breast cancer can help to put their own experience into perspective. Thoughts and feelings that had originally seemed aberrant become normalized and easier to accept (Spiegel, 1979). In the context of a group, the breast cancer patient discovers that her response is not exceptional but a normal reaction to an abnormal situation. The normalization of women's experiences makes it easier for each woman to consider how cancer has changed her. In listening to others, witnessing their tears, and sharing laughter at the absurdity of some of life's situations, she becomes more aware of the universal nature of her experience. Furthermore, the opportunity to share her ordeal enables her to work toward integrating these new aspects of her life into a stable and coherent self and body image.

GOALS OF SUPPORTIVE-EXPRESSIVE PSYCHOTHERAPY GROUPS

BUILDING BONDS

We are fundamentally social creatures, more like ants than eagles. From the moment of birth our survival is contingent upon our ability to engage others in caring for us. Our relative lack of size and strength in the animal kingdom is offset by our social skills—our ability to plan, remember, organize, and communicate. Our species has survived because of its ability to form social networks that provide for mutual support. Social support is an important mediating factor in dealing with stressful life events (Moos and Schaefer, 1987; Folkman and Lazarus, 1980; Wortman and Dunkel-Schetter, 1987; Dunkel-Schetter, Feinstein et al., 1992; Bloom and Spiegel, 1984).

Social networks provide a reservoir of instrumental assistance, relieving someone in the middle of a crisis of the need to carry out routine activities of daily living, or new activities required by an illness. They also supply a menu of alternative coping strategies, and more important, they offer role reinforcement for those immersed in an unwelcome situation: It is especially important to feel like a good mother or friend after being told you have cancer. Preserving domains of competence and self-esteem is critical during times when patients feel as though the rug has been pulled out from under them. Having cancer potentially threatens the ability to perform many roles. With each area of competence lost, the disease seems more pervasive and serious.

Conversely, the ability to help and be helped by others places boundaries on the ravages of disease. Thus, joining a support group can go a long way toward reducing the feelings of isolation, the sense of having been cut out of the herd, that often beset cancer patients (Spiegel, Bloom et al., 1981). The fact that all group members are facing the same disease becomes a powerful bonding force. Psychotherapy, especially in groups, provides a new social network composed of individuals facing similar problems (Yalom, 1995; Spiegel, 1994b). Just at a time when illness makes a person feel removed from the flow of life, psychotherapeutic support provides a new and important social connection.

There is strong evidence that social contact not only has positive emotional effects, but that it reduces overall mortality risk (House, Landis et al., 1988) as well as that from cancer (Reynolds and Kaplan, 1990). Indeed, social isolation has been shown to be as strongly related to age-adjusted mortality as are serum cholesterol levels or smoking. Being married predicts a better medical outcome with cancer (Goodwin, Hunt et al., 1987). Thus, constructing new social networks for cancer patients via support groups and other means is doubly important; it comes at a time when their natural social support from family and friends may have eroded and when more support is needed (Mulder, van der Pompe et al., 1992).

Attending a support group often allows members to relate to each other in special ways that counter the social isolation often experienced after a cancer diagnosis (Tracy and Gussow, 1976; Toseland and Hacker, 1982). Being part of a group can afford cancer patients a sense of community necessary for successful coping and provide opportunities to learn from each other. In a review of the social comparison literature, Taylor and Lobel (1989) observe that cancer patients seek interactions with other patients who have either overcome their illness or are adjusting well. This provides them with information about how to cope, examples which demonstrate that it can be done well, and a sense of belonging, a positive identity by affiliation with those who have an attribute that makes them feel excluded elsewhere.

Another social benefit of group support can be conceptualized as the helper-therapy principle (Riessman, 1965). Having cancer would seem to be a meaningless tragedy—no good would likely come from it. However, when a cancer patient has learned something about how to manage the disease and because of this can help someone else, then something genuinely good has emerged from a bad situation. The tragedy of having cancer is converted into an asset that enables one person to provide concrete help to another. Similarly, the patient develops a sense of competence in dealing with the illness to the extent that he or she can be of genuine help to others in a support group. Cancer patients find other patients to be most helpful when they model successful coping and surviving (Taylor and Dakof, 1988). Many newly recurrent cancer patients have reported that "it was helpful to discuss their concerns objectively with someone outside of their family" (Mahon, Cella et al., 1990, p. 51). Group therapy increases the likelihood of constructive compassion with other cancer patients (Yalom 1995). Therapy comes in the giving as well as the receiving. Thus, it may not come as a surprise that cancer patients also seek others who are adjusting poorly.

> In one of our groups that had been running for six years, a new member had recently joined. She was quite ill because of rapidly advancing disease and a bone marrow transplant. Group members discussed how vigorous and effective it made them feel as a group to be able to mobilize themselves to support her. Marion, a member who only came to the group once a month because of the three-hour drive to get there, added, "In some ways I barely know you. Our lives have just brushed by one another. Yet I consider you a real friend, and was so glad to be able to visit you in the hospital. It means a great deal to me to be able to see you through this." At a time when you would think a cancer patient has enough to do to keep existing family and friendship networks together, these cancer patients went out of their way to include new members and continue their group.

Being with others who have the same illness and who share similar experiences mitigates the anxiety of facing the illness alone and normalizes disease-related feelings and experiences. The type of isolation to which breast cancer patients are subjected is often experienced as a harbinger of death (Spiegel, 1990)—complete aloneness and separation from family and friends. Joining a support group can be an effective antidote to feelings of isolation (Yalom and Greaves, 1977; Spiegel and Yalom, 1978; Spiegel,

Bloom et al., 1981). A support group has the beneficial effect of moderating the sense of isolation by providing a new social network. The group becomes a powerful medium for restoring the patient's homeostasis in that the very experience that seems to separate her from the rest of the world is what bonds her with the group (Spiegel, 1990). Often group members find that little needs to be said in order to communicate what is going on for them. When times are difficult, each woman knows that the group will be there to support and understand her; and when the group ends, these friendships frequently continue. By virtue of being in the group, these women feel less alone and construct an important new network of social support.

> *Marie was only thirty-seven when she was diagnosed with inflammatory breast cancer, an especially aggressive tumor. She was an energetic, dramatic, and active woman, a beloved dance instructor, wife, and mother. She was jolted by the news and joined a support group soon after the diagnosis. This was, in fact, before her mastectomy, since, with inflammatory carcinoma, it is customary to give chemotherapy in hopes of shrinking the tumor prior to removing it. Thus, she had been in the group for about six weeks before the operation. One of the women from the group came to the hospital to be with her on the day of the surgery. When Marie returned some weeks later, she commented: "You know, your visit meant more to me than anyone else's that day, because you knew exactly what I was going through."*

This observation of Marie's would seem quite surprising. That a relative stranger's visit should mean more than that of her husband, daughters, and close friends seems counterintuitive. Yet, at such moments, a certain kind of understanding can come from someone in the same boat that is different from the support provided by loved ones. One is not necessarily better or more important than the other: They are different. The support that develops in such groups is intense, and grows rapidly. Unlike traditional group therapy, in which relationships in the group are a dry run for those in real life (Yalom, 1995), the affiliations formed in such support groups are real, new sources of emotional sustenance.

EXPRESSING EMOTIONS

Psychotherapy groups are a powerful social laboratory, providing a means whereby the here-and-now can be used to try out interpersonal skills, to test how one person comes across to another or how a problem or situation sounds to others. Yalom (1995) describes the key element of intensive psychotherapy groups as working in the "here-and-now," but from a similar dual perspective: "The here-and-now focus, to be effective, consists of two symbiotic tiers, neither of which has therapeutic power without the other" (p. 129). The first involves paying primary attention to immediate events occurring within the group: "The immediate events in the meeting take precedence over events both in the current outside life and in the distant past of the members" (1995, p. 129). This may seem paradoxical in a group devoted to helping people with the effects of serious illness: real-life events. Certainly the common basis for involvement is the occurrence of similar real-life problems. Yet it is the impact of these problems on the life of the group that is the key focus: The *we* of the group takes precedence over the *I* of each member. Disappointments and losses become group problems rather than a series of individual problems. They are thus managed collectively rather than individually. Furthermore, Yalom emphasizes that "illumination of process" (1995) is the other key element of this kind of group work: observation as well as participation. To be effective, good psychotherapy groups must not merely be *present*; they must simultaneously be *reflective*. The most intense aspect of this group modeling is the expression of emotion.

Support and expression of feeling reinforce each other. Providing an atmosphere in which the expression of all emotion is encouraged is a critical task of therapists. Their job is to follow the affect, more so than tracking the content or completing stories. This conveys to patients that the group is a place where their distress can be expressed and addressed.

Andrea knew that her breast cancer was advancing. She had liver involvement and could feel herself becoming sicker week by week. She began talking about assisted suicide in her group: "I'm just a burden to my family now—they'd be better off without me," she told the group. We knew a good deal about her family, and could easily have taken the path of speculating about how they felt about her and her thoughts of ending her life. But we took a different tack. The leader said, "I think Andrea is posing a question to us, and I would like us to answer it for her. Would we be better off if she were not here? Is she a burden to us?" "It means so much to me to see you every week," said Debra. "I have learned so much from you—from watching you change. You are so different now—so much more direct. I want you here." Others chimed in with similar sentiments. Andrea could hear and feel her importance to the group, with the obvious analogy to her family's feelings. She died peacefully without artificial assistance several months later.

Thus, groups have a special tool at their disposal: the use of the immediate group process as a means of examining real relationships and trying out interaction patterns for other relationships in life. Harry Stack Sullivan (Sullivan, 1953) defined psychotherapy as "participant-observation," meaning that the relationship (in his case, the therapist-patient relationship in individual psychotherapy) must be real enough that patient and therapist care about each other, but never so intimate that one cannot step back and observe, learning what is going on in the relationship and why. Group psychotherapy contains an even stronger dose of participation—real relationships are built that extend outside the group room—but it works as a therapy because everything is open to examination; patients talk about how they feel about each other and learn a great deal in the process.

A group for women with metastatic breast cancer was painfully discussing its first loss. Donna had died quite suddenly. She and her husband had planned a trip to Hawaii. Instead, she was hospitalized and died several days later. There was a palpable sense of shock. The overt discussion involved the sense of unfinished business—no one had a chance to say good-bye, or to prepare emotionally for the loss. It was experienced as a shock to the group. At another level, it stimulated death anxiety in everyone. Members had been living with an unwritten rule: There would be warning. One would know and have time to plan when the end was in sight. But this death violated that unspoken rule, and made everyone doubly anxious. The discussion of loss was parsed into components: Not only had Donna died, she had died suddenly. The group had immediate work to do: grieving. But it also had to make sense of the loss, reflect on its unique as well as its general elements. This led to a recognition in the group that preparation for death was crucial, indeed soothing. Death could be better faced and managed when it did not seem like a sneak attack. The group learned by counterexample what it hoped for in a "good" death.

Thus, the examination of group process in the here-and-now deepened the examination of grief and death anxiety, and led to a means of coping. By directly facing the most painful aspects of the loss, it was possible to emerge from the discussion with a plan for mitigating the potential damage done by death: Greater attention to the process of dying as well as the fact of death could cushion its blow.

Openness and emotional expressiveness are central goals of supportive-expressive group treatment. Indeed, they are the reason for the use of the word *expressive*. Patients often feel pressure to appear strong and act as though they were more able to cope with their situation than in fact they feel. Yet these attempts to hide their real emotions and display a positive attitude are ineffective and can consume a great deal of emotional energy. Furthermore, many people with cancer unwittingly make a kind of devil's bargain. In their efforts to suppress "negative" affect, they tend to suppress all emotion, for fear of letting go of the control that suppresses dysphoria. Group members often discover that after they have had a good cry, they can have a good laugh as well.

After a painful discussion regarding the burden of making plans for the burial of their remains, Muriel talked about her recent experience in calling a local cemetery and asking what it would cost her to be buried there. She was doing this to spare her family the painful task of making these arrangements. She was quoted an astronomical price for a burial plot, so she reported having said, "Actually, I represent a group of women who are looking for a place to be buried." There was a long pause on the phone, and then the woman replied: "Skylawn Park does not offer group discounts." Everyone in the group had a good laugh over this ultimate attempt at bargaining.

Even a shy or reticent group member can gain a lot from participation. Observing what others gain can teach a great deal—members can benefit by identification. However, Yalom (1995) cautions that prolonged silence usually does not bode well: It is a communication of noninvolvement, an unwillingness to take risks and participate with others, which may affect the group as a whole, and not just the silent member. Nonetheless, in the short run, relatively uninvolved patients may be drawn in to supportive-expressive groups, encouraged to become involved gradually. In many ways this process can be more natural and unhurried than in individual therapy or counseling, where little of use will occur if the patient has little to say.

A major goal of supportive-expressive group therapy is to help group members to express all emotions, whether they are "negative" or "positive." In this way they should not be hiding or denying any salient aspect of their experience. If negative affect is not allowed expression, a great deal of energy is required to suppress or bypass it. With its free expression, group members experience relief and obtain encouragement as they find that they are able to tolerate it. Indeed, the dysphoria seems less overwhelming: "I am more than my problems and fears," one patient concluded. As group members find that their emotions are better tolerated by both themselves and their group, they develop the courage to be more open and expressive with their loved ones as well.

Detoxifying Death and Dying

Thoughts of death and dying provoke deep fear in all of us, but, for the most part, we can effectively put them aside. When stricken with a potentially life-threatening disease, however, the fear is gripping and unavoidable. Even so, patients usually try to avoid these topics. Typically their avoidance is reinforced at home or by friends who feel uncomfortable talking about the possibility of their loved ones dying. The result is that patients are left alone with their terrifying fantasies—patients and families suffer separately rather than together. Without someone or someplace where they can unveil and look at these fearful images, the underlying anxiety will maintain its stranglehold on their emotional state.

Being consciously or unconsciously gripped by anxiety and fear about dying adversely affects a person's ability to embrace life and live it fully. By helping the patient tolerate her thoughts of death and dying, we have in a sense "detoxified" the thoughts; their potency and ability to detract from living diminishes.

Diane, who had metastatic breast cancer and experienced considerable pain, made up her mind to fulfill a lifelong dream by traveling to Santa Fe for the opera. At first she had thought the cancer would prevent her from going. She decided that even though the cancer was inescapable, she was going to the opera anyway. Initially she had thought of the threat as an impediment to going because the experience would be difficult and less than perfect. With the help of the group, however, she began to think of it differently. "Who knows how many more chances I will have to go to the opera there?" she mused. "So I brought my cancer with me. It sat in the seat next to me. But I loved the opera." The group congratulated her on having made the trip. They viewed it as an inspiration to them to do likewise. The story, like their lives, was not perfect, but it was what they had, and they determined to make the most of it.

Grace, another group member, had given up a successful technical career to study art. She brought in a painting of herself that expressed two perspectives—as she saw herself

now, and as she had been when young. The first image was larger, in strong flesh tones;
the latter more slender and remote, in a dusky blue. She called the painting Regret. In
describing the painting Grace talked about her changed body image and the effects of ag-
ing. "But," the therapist commented, "the 'older' body image seems much more alive."
Grace was a bit shocked, but then smiled and said, "I had not thought of that, but it is
true. My body now is not perfect, but it is very much alive. In fact, I feel more comfort-
able about enjoying my body now than I did when I was younger." Thus, in the group
process members are encouraged to distinguish vitality from perfection, living fully
from the threat of death.

Helping the patient break a threatening subject down into more manageable pieces has the effect of reducing the terror associated with the topic. It
comes to seem very real indeed, but less overwhelming because it can be
faced. In this sense, we think of death as being detoxified. By addressing
death and related problems directly, the fear and anxiety will eventually decrease (Spiegel and Glafkides, 1983; Spiegel, Bloom et al., 1981). Naturally,
simply raising the topic immediately elicits fear and anxiety, but, by facing
her worst fears openly and directly, the patient will find that not only can
she can tolerate these thoughts but that there are actually things she can do
to lessen her anxiety. Often patients experience relief simply because they
are able to talk about their anxiety openly, converting a generalized dread
into specific fears.

Some discover that one of their fears is of dying a painful death and that
they can ease their anxiety about this by writing a living will describing how
they want others to care for them if that situation arises. The aim is not to
make the fear and anxiety go away, for that is surely an impossibility, but
rather to make the topic of death and dying something patients can tolerate
and deal with (Spiegel and Yalom, 1978; Spiegel, 1993b). The topic may still
be disturbing but at least it can be addressed.

You may have noted that this approach is quite different from many of the
mind/body approaches to emotional support proffered to cancer patients in
books and magazine articles. Our emphasis is not on cultivating a "positive"
attitude, but rather on developing realistic optimism, finding those aspects
of life that are controllable and making the most of them, while accepting
those parts of the disease that are inevitable. Hope is always important, but
it is really a question of hope for what: a long life or a good life? We urge our
patients to hope for the best but prepare for the worst.

REDEFINING LIFE PRIORITIES

Cancer produces an uncertain future. However, the possibility of a fore-shortened future has the effect of focusing attention on vital issues. There is often a sense of urgency about defining life goals or in reaching goals already set. Similarly, we try to cultivate impatience with issues felt to be trivial or distracting. "Cancer cures neurosis," Irvin Yalom is fond of saying. The aim is to help each patient develop and refine a life project. This involves achieving clarity of life values and goals, as well as to best use limited resources of time and energy.

Discussions of life goals can be an important way of helping patients restructure the impact of the illness on their lives. It forces an evaluation of life values and a recognition that putting off important goals until a later time simply will not do, because a later time may be too late. Often this enables patients to develop new goals and sometimes discover that they want to live and enjoy life more fully in the present (Spiegel and Yalom, 1978). It is important that patients realize that the time left may be short, although it's not an inevitability. Consequently, they are encouraged to use this precious time well. The diagnosis presents these women with the opportunity and motivation to do something that we all would benefit from doing.

INCREASING THE SUPPORT
OF FRIENDS AND FAMILY

Psychotherapeutic interventions can be quite helpful in repairing existing relationships outside the group: improving communication, getting needs met, increasing role flexibility, and adjusting to new medical, social, vocational, and financial realities. The atmosphere of openness and support cultivated in groups can usefully spread to the family as well. There is evidence that open and shared problem solving in families results in reduced anxiety and depression in cancer patients (Spiegel, Bloom et al., 1983; Friedman, Baer et al., 1988; Gritz, Wellisch et al., 1990). Exploration in the group therapy setting provides a model for similar openness at home, helping members identify problems and anticipating the results of their greater openness. Thus, facilitating open exploration of common problems is an important therapeutic goal.

Patients and families often try to spare each other by avoiding difficult topics (Lewis and Hammond, 1992). Unfortunately, this occurs at a time when the patient needs all the support she can get. Family members can be a significant source of emotional and practical help to the patient. It is important that the patient be able to make full use of that resource. The aim is to help the patient identify the kind of support she wants and can expect from those around her, as well as learn how to ask for what she needs. This process can be facilitated in the group by helping members to clarify their own needs and wants and developing the ability to ask those around them for the support they desire.

The ultimate goal is to improve communication between patients and their families and friends. Participation in supportive-expressive groups is designed to encourage open and honest communication with family members. This includes learning to express anxieties, wishes, and fears without excessive concern about protecting the family from worry. At the same time, the group should encourage receptiveness on the part of the patient to hearing the concerns of others, both in the group and in the family, allowing others to communicate openly as well. Members of the group can reflect feelings that family members would have in a given situation: "If I were your husband, I wouldn't know what to do right now to help you. Perhaps that is part of why he is such a disappointment to you in this crisis" is one example of such an intervention. In reducing barriers created by fear and concern, patients can make full use of their social support system and in so doing find a source of sustenance to carry them through the cancer experience (Spiegel, Bloom et al., 1983).

Improving the Doctor–Patient Relationship

The quality of the patient's relationship with her physician is vital and unfortunately is often less than ideal. Patients frequently struggle with it: "Am I getting the information I need? Is it okay to be phoning my doctor for every new ache and pain? My doctor seems so busy, I feel I'm not getting the attention I need."

Thus, another goal of the group is to help frequently develop good working relationships with their doctors, with more active participation on the patients' part. In the current medical system the doctor is often seen as someone not to be questioned. This situation does not lead to a productive doctor–patient relationship. Instead, patients need to move from a passive stance to a more active one. Rather than being a dependent recipient of treatment, the patient should be a partner in the treatment.

This process involves improving communication between patients and doctors so that patients are able to state what they want and need from their physicians, to ask questions, and to be involved in treatment decisions. A group member will express concern about some new ache or pain. "When is your next appointment with your doctor?" another group member asks. "In a month," is the response. "Don't wait that long," she is told. "Why should you worry about it for a whole month? See your doctor tomorrow." Group members frequently encourage one another to participate more actively in their health care, sometimes to the point of accompanying them to their doctors' offices.

When confronted with a potentially lethal disease such as cancer, patients often feel helpless, powerless, and uncomfortably dependent upon physicians, nurses, and other health care providers. Our goal is to help these patients identify their own needs and devise a plan of action to meet them. Part of this is learning how to develop a true partnership with physicians in managing their health care; to be able to ask for the support they need from family and friends; and to make active choices about treatment, daily activities, and life goals.

IMPROVING COPING SKILLS

The classical literature on coping (Folkman and Lazarus, 1980; Moos and Schaefer, 1987) describes three fundamental types of coping: information-focused, emotion-focused, and problem-focused. Most medical intervention is directed at the first only: enhancing information-focused coping by telling patients what is wrong with them, what their prognosis is, and what their treatment will be. Unfortunately, this does not address the strong emotional reactions patients have to the information given them, reactions that may impair their ability to take in new information.

Furthermore, passivity in the face of threat only reinforces helplessness. For example, a recent study of genetic counseling for women at high genetic risk for breast and ovarian cancer (BrCA1 gene) found that while the provision of genetic information helped, many women continued to misperceive their risk of cancer after the counseling, especially those who were highly anxious (Lerman, Lustbader et al., 1995). Indeed, the most anxious women got the least from the genetic counseling. This form of coping has an element of passivity to it as well: The patient is the recipient of information, but there often seems to be little the patient can do about this new knowledge. Patients respond better to any problem when they can find a way to take a more active stance toward it. They are comforted by their participation in treatment, by the feeling that they are doing something to counter the illness.

Patients with cancer are confronted with all kinds of new situations and problems. Most feel unprepared to deal with these new demands. There are issues about how to deal with relationships with family, friends, co-workers, and physicians. Everything has shifted both within patients' images of themselves and in how others relate to them. Coping strategies that once worked in the past no longer seem relevant or appropriate. Our goal is to help cancer patients expand and improve their repertoire of coping skills. One major source of inspiration is hearing how others have learned to cope in similar situations. By learning from each other in this way, patients are often able to expand their domain of coping skills, expanding their knowledge of alternatives and their willingness to try them.

Since affect is often an obstacle to obtaining and acting on information, developing an ability to recognize, tolerate, and express uncomfortable affect is an important part of supportive-expressive group therapy, as discussed above. This allows patients to progress from the receptive mode of gaining information to managing also the affect that the information elicits. This enables the information to sink in, as a variety of feelings associated with it emerge. Following this working through of emotion, patients can come to the more active mode of resolving difficulties: problem-focused coping.

One specific coping mechanism we teach is self-hypnosis (Spiegel and Spiegel, 1987). Hypnosis is a simple form of highly focused attention (absorption), something like looking through a telephoto lens. What you see is visible in great detail, but it is devoid of context. This experience of focused attention is coupled with physical relaxation, an ability to put out of awareness things normally in consciousness (dissociation), and heightened sensitivity to social cues (suggestibility). Self-hypnosis is a skill that patients can use to help them better manage pain (Spiegel and Bloom, 1983a; Hilgard and Hilgard, 1975; Brose and Spiegel, 1992; Spiegel, 1985), overcome sleep disturbance, and reduce stress and anxiety (Lang and Joyce, 1996). It is also a strategy that can be used to consolidate perspectives gained from group interaction, put new problems into perspective, and consider alternative ways of coping.

Betty thought she had come to terms with her own breast cancer, diagnosed a year earlier. But she felt herself disintegrating when she learned that her beloved husband had Alzheimer's disease. She felt imprisoned by the unwelcome information, as though she had just emerged from one catastrophe only to be hit by one that seemed far worse. She cried as she pictured what lay ahead for herself and her husband.

She was asked to use a familiar self-hypnosis exercise to picture this tragedy on an imaginary screen, divided in two. On one half, she pictured their decline together with great sadness and apprehension. Then she was asked to picture on the other half of the screen what she wanted: "To go down with love," she replied, with some surprise. She emerged feeling she had a plan, a goal that would make the remainder of their lives together meaningful. The hypnosis exercise allowed her to turn inward, tolerate the anxiety and sadness that accompanied her situation, and find some aspect of it she could do something about. Although many think of hypnosis as a state of being controlled, it is actually a means of teaching people how to enhance their sense of control over stressful situations. This method and how it was used to help Betty is discussed in more detail in Chapter 11.

In summary, attaining the goals described above will lead to an enhanced quality of life: more intense and meaningful relationships, clearer priorities, and greater authenticity in living. Quality of life is vastly improved by an effective social support system that is open to emotional expression, provides help as needed, receives as well as gives, and where there is role flexibility. The sense of isolation and aloneness is diminished. There is a feeling of taking charge as patients feel able to ask for what they need and have clarity about what they want to accomplish in their lives. Even though they may not be able to control the course of the disease, they grow from being able to better control the life the disease leaves to them. These groups help cancer patients mourn their losses, bear uncomfortable feelings, solidify social support, and take charge of their treatment and the remainder of their lives. Supportive-expressive therapy groups acknowledge the reality of how uncomfortable it is to be a cancer patient, and use this common plight as a basis for building new and more effective means of coping with the stress of the illness. We now turn to the literature examining evidence of the need for as well as the effectiveness of supportive-expressive and other types of support groups for the medically ill.

EVIDENCE FOR THE BENEFITS OF PSYCHOTHERAPEUTIC INTERVENTIONS

PSYCHOLOGICAL AND SOCIAL RESULTS

Many studies have shown positive effects of group therapy interventions for cancer patients (Fawzy, 1991; Fawzy, Fawzy et al., 1995; Ferlic, Goldman et al., 1979; Gustafson and Whitman, 1978; Wood, Milligan et al., 1978; Spiegel, Bloom et al., 1981; Spiegel and Bloom, 1983; Anderson, 1992). Psychosocial interventions have proven efficacious in helping breast cancer patients to better cope with the illness and live more fully (Turns, 1988). There is now clear evidence that various psychotherapies for cancer patients affect specific symptoms, for example, reducing anxiety and depression (Ferlic, Goldman et al., 1979; Gustafson and Whitman, 1978; Wood, Milligan et al., 1978; Spiegel, Bloom et al., 1981; Spiegel and Bloom, 1983; Mulder, van der Pompe et al., 1992), improving coping skills (Turns, 1988; Fawzy, Cousins et al., 1990), and reducing pain, nausea, and vomiting (Forester, Kornfeld et al., 1985; Cain, Kohorn et al., 1986; Morrow and Morrell, 1982). Indeed, group therapy is now recommended as a component of standard treatment for breast cancer (Henderson, Garber et al., 1990).

In a thorough review of the psychosocial intervention literature with cancer patients, Fawzy and colleagues (1995) find generally positive results, with improvements cited across four general types of intervention: education, behavioral training, individual psychotherapy, and group psychotherapy. They recommend a rather structured intervention for recently diagnosed patients, arguing that such an approach is easily promulgated and is less stigmatizing than more exploratory, less structured psychotherapeutic approaches:

> A structured, psychiatric intervention consisting of health education, stress management and behavioral training, coping including problem-solving techniques, and psychosocial group support offers the greatest potential benefit for patients who are newly diagnosed or in the early stages of their treatment. Patients are usually distressed, anxious and unable to effectively utilize their normal coping styles. . . . The advantages of such a program include easy implementation and replication, promotion of important

illness-related problem-solving skills, and increased participation in decision making and active coping. A short-term, structured, psychoeducational group intervention is the model that we propose to be used for newly diagnosed patients and/or patients with good prognoses. The focus is on learning how to live with cancer (Fawzy, Fawzy et al., 1995, p. 112).

They go on to recommend our supportive-expressive model for patients with advanced disease: "We also encourage the development of ongoing weekly group support programs for patients with advanced metastatic disease, based on the studies of Spiegel et al., that focus on daily coping, pain management, and dealing with the existential issues related to death and dying" (Fawzy, Fawzy et al., 1995, p. 112). The point of view espoused by Dr. Fawzy is one that merits further research. Our initial findings with women with primary breast cancer indicate that a more exploratory, affect-arousing intervention is effective with women with primary disease (Spiegel, Morrow et al., 1996) as well as advanced cancer, although it seems to be most advantageous for the more distressed patients (Classen, Koopman et al., in submission). One of the future challenges of this field is to better delineate specific methods applicable to specific populations.

Trijsburg and colleagues (Trijsburg, van Knippenberg et al., 1992) systematically reviewed twenty-two controlled trials of psychological treatment for cancer patients. They found evidence for the effectiveness of these interventions in nineteen of the twenty-two studies, leading them to conclude that psychological treatment is beneficial. However, they felt the evidence was not clear regarding the possible superiority of group over individual intervention (p. 510). They compared results with three types of intervention: "tailored," meaning more open-ended psychotherapies that tailored the treatment to the patient problems presented; "structured counseling" interventions, which were more psychoeducational in nature; and "behavioral interventions and hypnosis." They found that the tailored interventions were especially effective in reducing overall distress, improving self-concept, and improving health locus of control, but there was less evidence for specific reductions in anxiety and depression. The structured counseling interventions showed specific efficacy in reducing depression.

The behavioral interventions were designed to reduce pain, nausea, and vomiting and were effective in this regard. However, they also demonstrated effectiveness in reducing anxiety. They noted that while many of the interventions tested were minimalist in nature, designed to provide as little intervention as necessary, there were quite good results with longer interventions: "Although the development of cost-effective and less time-consuming interventions may appear attractive in a number of respects, intensive and long-term counseling yields significant changes in several essential functional areas. Therefore, it would be appropriate to study the differential effects of (spaced-out) long-term counseling and short-term interventions. Longer follow-up periods, extending over several years, could yield important findings concerning adaptation and survival" (p. 514). Thus, in this review there is evidence that psychotherapeutic treatment for cancer patients works, and that more of it may be better, especially for those with advanced disease.

Krupnick and colleagues (1993) reach a similar conclusion: "There is virtually unanimous agreement that group participation facilitates psychological adaptation. More recently, provocative data have suggested that such participation also may affect physical adaptation, and, for some patients, might extend survival time" (p. 278). They attempt to match models of treatment with stage of disease, recommending, similar to the Fawzy (1995) review cited above, that earlier in the course of disease the interventions be more formal and psychoeducational, while later in the disease, more affectively expressive and long-term group interventions be encouraged. This overall approach is consistent with the model presented in this book, except that we recommend affective expression even in early-stage groups.

In our own studies, supportive-expressive group psychotherapy has proven to be quite effective in reducing dysphoria and improving adjustment to cancer. We (Spiegel, Bloom et al., 1981; Spiegel and Bloom, 1983; Spiegel, Bloom et al., 1989) undertook a prospective study on the effect of psychosocial intervention on quality of life and survival time of eighty-six patients with metastatic breast cancer in the 1970s. These patients met on a weekly basis for ninety-minute sessions of supportive-expressive group therapy. Patients were evaluated in this randomized study for mood disturbance, tension-anxiety, fatigue, confusion, pain reduction, and survival time. The group focused on problems of terminal illness, including improving relationships with family, friends, and physicians, and living as fully as possible in the face of death.

The patients were tested at four-month intervals, and the treatment group was found to have lower levels of mood disturbance, fewer maladaptive coping responses, and fewer phobic responses than the control group

(Spiegel, Bloom et al., 1981). Indeed, treatment patients improved in mood over the course of the year, while control patients worsened. After patients in the treatment group were taught self-hypnosis techniques, they had half the pain of those in the control group at the end of the initial study year (Spiegel and Bloom, 1983a). Although the frequency and duration of pain did not differentiate the groups, the treatment groups experienced less discomfort and intensity of pain. An analysis of the content and affect in fourteen support group sessions demonstrated that the deterioration or death of a member affected the content of the groups but not their affective quality (Spiegel and Glafkides, 1983), leading them to conclude that these groups do not demoralize members.

We are currently conducting an intervention trial with a new sample of 125 metastatic breast cancer patients. In this study we are again assessing the psychosocial and survival benefits of participating in long-term supportive-expressive group psychotherapy. It is too soon for us to know whether being in the treatment group has affected survival in this sample. However, we have examined the effect of treatment on psychological distress and found that women who were in the treatment group were significantly less distressed one year after entering the study compared to the women assigned to the control condition (Classen, Butler et al., in submission).

We have also conducted studies of similar support groups for women with recently diagnosed breast cancer. In collaboration with the Community Clinical Oncology Program of the National Cancer Institute, we trained two therapists, at each of eleven busy oncology practices in the United States, to run a twelve-week program of group support. Typically these were oncology nurses and psychologists. Our preliminary findings are that the groups reduced anxiety and depression, as the more extensive groups had for women with metastatic disease (Spiegel, Morrow et al., 1996). Analysis of more extensive data from a randomized trial indicates that brief supportive-expressive group therapy was most beneficial for those women who were initially high in mood disturbance (Classen, Koopman et al., in submission).

This treatment model, supportive-expressive group psychotherapy (Spiegel, Bloom et al., 1989; Spiegel, 1993b), has been compared in a randomized prospective trial to cognitive/behavioral treatment in a sample of HIV-infected patients (Kelly, Murphy et al., 1993). This more emotionally expressive approach was found to be more effective in reducing mood disturbance.

Many of the psychotherapies that have shown promise in improving emotional adjustment, and have even influenced survival time, involve encouraging open expression of emotion and assertiveness in assuming control over the course of treatment, life decisions, and relationships (Spiegel, Bloom et al., 1981, 1989; Fawzy, Cousins et al., 1990; Fawzy, Fawzy et al., 1993, 1995; Spiegel and Yalom, 1978). While belief that one has control over the cause of a disease leads to poor outcome, belief in control over the course of the disease leads to better outcome (Watson, Pruyn et al., 1990).

Overall we have found that the kind of direct and caring confrontation with the issues surrounding anxiety about disease progression, dying, and death that occurs in these groups does far more good than harm. One metastatic breast cancer patient who had participated in a weekly support group for five years comments, "This group is the least superficial thing I do in my life."

ADHERENCE WITH MEDICAL TREATMENT

Another potential benefit of psychosocial intervention is improvement of patients' cooperation with their physicians and their medical treatment. Adherence with the treatment regimen, defined as the match between the patient's behavior and health care advice (Haynes, Taylor et al., 1979), is important because better adherence may prolong disease-free and overall survival (Motzer, Geller et al., 1990; Hoagland, Morrow et al., 1983; Steckel, 1982; Harris, Lippman et al., 1992; Richardson, Shelton et al., 1990).

Adherence issues may be particularly important for cancer treatment regimens, due to their complexity, intensity, and side effects. Despite this fact, there has been little systematic research on adherence with treatment among cancer patients (Given and Given, 1989). The existing data suggest that nonadherence to treatment regimens is high among cancer patients. In one study, 23 percent of patients did not keep their appointments for the administration of chemotherapy (Itano, Tanabe et al., 1983b). Withdrawal from the recommended treatment protocol is estimated to range from 16 to 33 percent (Glass, Wieand et al., 1981; Laszlo and Lucas, 1981; Lee, 1983; Wilcox, Fetting et al., 1982).

In a study of women with abnormal Pap smears requiring follow-up care, 29 percent did not return for screening follow-up (Marcus, Crane et al., 1992). In another survey, 246 randomly selected oncologists (Hoagland, Morrow et al., 1983) reported that the most frequent adherence problem was failure to return following initial evaluation for the recommended outpatient treatment. Other major problems included failure to keep subsequent appointments, patient refusal of the recommended inpatient and/or outpatient treatments, and nonadherence with the prescribed home medication regimen (Itano, Tanabe et al., 1983b).

Thus, even in the life-threatening situation of cancer, cooperation with medical treatment is anything but uniform. Variables that have been shown to affect adherence include demographics; patient perceptions of their illness and their role in its treatment; social support; the costs and benefits of adherence from the patient's perspective; and an intention to comply (Given and Given, 1989). All of these psychosocial factors (except demographics) may be influenced by involvement in a cancer support group. Participating in a group increases patients' knowledge, changes their attitudes about treatment, and may help them overcome practical obstacles to adherence. Other factors, such as educating patients about the efficacy of treatments, can produce better adherence with medication regimens (Ferguson and Bole, 1979; Beck, Parker et al., 1988). To the extent that groups help patients take an active and collaborative role in their medical treatment, there will be greater satisfaction and adherence (Eisenthal, Emery et al., 1979; Wyszynski, 1990).

There is reason to predict that participation in supportive-expressive therapy groups will improve adherence by helping patients to (1) better manage the anxiety that is interwoven with treatment, (2) better comprehend the reasoning behind treatment decisions, (3) feel more in control of the course of their treatment through clearer communication with their physicians, and (4) more effectively mobilize support from family and friends for participating in treatment.

COST-EFFECTIVENESS

Group therapy is clearly more cost-effective than individual therapy in that it makes limited professional resources available to many more patients, including underserved populations. Economically, group therapy may be up to four times more affordable for patients and for institutions (Hellman, Budd et al., 1990; Yalom, 1995; Yalom and Yalom, 1990). Several well-conducted meta-analytic studies have illuminated a large literature demonstrating that psychoeducational (Devine, 1992) and psychotherapeutic (Mumford, Schlesinger et al., 1984; Strain, Lyons et al., 1991) interventions produce cost-savings in medical treatment.

Effects on medical practice resulting from such psychosocial interventions for medically ill patient populations include more rapid recovery from surgery (Devine, 1992), shorter hospital stays (Devine, 1992; Mumford, Schlesinger et al., 1984; Strain, Lyons et al., 1991), and reduced distress-related outpatient visits to doctors (Cummings and VandenBos, 1981; Lorig, Lubeck et al., 1985; Browne, Arpin, et al., 1990). This may seem surprising, but it can be understood in the context of research showing that a major reason for high utilization of medical services is poor adjustment to illness (Browne, Arpin et al., 1990) and co-morbid psychiatric conditions such as depressive and anxiety disorders (Von Korff, Ormel et al., 1992). Thus, means of addressing patient distress is of utmost importance to health care service delivery and cost considering the prevalence of adjustment problems among the medically ill.

STRESS AND HEALTH STATUS

While the primary and expected benefits of group therapy for the medically ill (including reduced distress) are psychosocial, more active coping, and better personal and professional relationships, there is reason to consider the possibility that living better might also mean living longer. There are adverse health effects of stress, and there is also evidence of positive effects of social support, including group intervention, on disease progression. While this is an area in need of substantial further research before any firm conclusions can be drawn, there is enough evidence now that it merits review.

Social stress such as divorce, loss of a job, or bereavement is associated with a greater likelihood of a relapse of cancer. The recent literature on stressful life events and cancer has developed in response to a study by Ramirez and colleagues (Ramirez, Craig et al., 1989) where they matched women with breast cancer that had recurred to a sample that remained disease-free. The relapsed group had experienced significantly more major life stress, such as bereavement and loss of jobs. For example, the frequency of family deaths or job loss among the relapsed patients yielded a relative risk of 5.67 compared to nonrecurrent breast cancer patients. This means that those with the most stressful lives had more than a fivefold greater risk of having a recurrence of breast cancer compared to those with the least stressful lives.

Barraclough and colleagues (Barraclough, Pinder et al., 1992; Barraclough, Osmond et al., 1993) followed 204 newly diagnosed breast cancer patients for 42 months after diagnosis and initial treatment. No relationship was found between stressful life events and risk of disease progression. The authors note that this was a limited follow-up time, but observed higher rates of bereavement in the nonrelapsing group. However, other studies have supported the observation of Ramirez and colleagues.

Geyer (1991) interviewed ninety-two women with undiagnosed breast lumps prior to diagnostic surgery regarding stressful life events during the previous eight years. Those women later determined to have a malignancy ($N = 33$) had experienced more stressful events than did women with benign tumors. Threat and loss were related to the likelihood of a malignancy independently of but as strongly as age. Both Barraclough's and Geyer's studies were prospective to some degree, but differ in that the dependent variable for the Barraclough study (like that for the Ramirez study) was recurrence, while that for the Geyer study was incidence, which could account for the apparently contradictory findings.

A study similar to Geyer's was conducted among malignant melanoma patients. Havlik and colleagues (Havlik, Vukasin et al., 1992) recruited fifty-six stage I and II melanoma patients into a retrospective study of stressful life events prior to diagnosis. A control group of fifty-six general surgery patients was randomly selected from hospital records. Telephone interviews were conducted with all participants to investigate the incidence within the last five years of divorce/separation, bankruptcy/unemployment of major wage earner, or death of a spouse/immediate family member. The melanoma patients had experienced significantly more stressful life events. While the issue is not completely resolved, and better conducted prospective studies at both points in the natural history of the disease are needed, three of these four studies indicate a relationship between stress and cancer.

SOCIAL RELATIONSHIP EFFECTS ON HEALTH STATUS

Social support can be conceptualized as a stress buffer, helping the individual absorb and manage the consequence of stressors, disease-related and otherwise. Recent research provides growing evidence for a modulating effect of social relationships on health. While this may seem surprising, keep in mind that we are fundamentally social creatures. From infancy, our survival depends on our social skills. Furthermore, social support and stress influence physiological systems, which affect the body's ability to fight disease, including the endocrine (Levine, Coe et al., 1989; McEwen, 1998; Van Cauter, Leproult et al., 1996), immune (Glaser, Kiecolt-Glaser et al., 1985, 1998; Glaser and Kiecolt-Glaser, 1986; Cohen, Tyrrell et al., 1991), and autonomic nervous systems (Cacioppo, 1994).

The evidence of social effects on health is actually quite clear. Social isolation elevates the risk of mortality from all causes as much as are high serum cholesterol levels or smoking (House, Landis et al., 1988). Decreased survival has been found to be associated with low quantity or quality of social relationships in several prospective studies (Rodin, 1986; House, Robbins et al., 1982; House, Lepkowski et al., 1994; Funch and Marshall, 1983; Goodwin, Hunt et al., 1987; Joffres, Reed et al., 1985; Ganster and Victor, 1988; Kennedy, Kiecolt-Glaser et al., 1988; Berkman and Syme, 1979).

This is not just a general relationship, but applies specifically to cancer-related mortality. Reynolds and Kaplan (1990) examined data on 6,928 adults and found that women who were socially isolated were at substantially elevated risk for dying of cancer. Those who had few social contacts and felt isolated had an almost twofold increase in incidence and a fivefold increase in relative risk for mortality from hormone-related cancers. Another clear example of the effect of social support on cancer progression is the finding that married cancer patients survive longer than unmarried persons (Goodwin, Hunt et al., 1987). Emotional support is associated with longer survival following a diagnosis of breast, colorectal, or lung cancer (Ell, Nishimoto et al., 1992). Of 294 patients studied, 74 had died. The majority (57 percent) of those had been diagnosed with breast cancer. They found that emotional support had a protective influence in regard to survival for patients with earlier stages of disease, especially among women with breast cancer. There was no effect with more advanced disease or among patients with lung or colorectal cancer. However, the limited number of patients among the latter two groups may have limited the capacity to detect relationships.

Waxler-Morrison and colleagues (1991) studied 133 patients diagnosed with primary intraductal breast cancer, of whom 26 had died at four-year follow-up and 38 had recurred. Utilizing the Cox Proportional Hazards Model, which is a method for analyzing predictions of survival time, they found that six of eleven measures of social relationships were significantly associated with longer survival. These were marital status; support from friends; contact with friends; total support from friends, relatives, and neighbors; employment status; and social network size. In particular, expressive-social activities and social support, not merely extroversion, were related to longer survival time.

Maunsell and colleagues (1995) studied 224 women with newly diagnosed breast cancer and examined the relationship between social support and mortality. Married women had a relative death rate of 0.86 compared to unmarried women over a seven-year follow-up. In contrast to women who had no confidants in the few months after surgery, those who did had a relative death rate of 0.55, and it was even lower among those who used more than one. Thus the availability of social support proved to be a robust predictor of subsequent mortality.

This literature provides clear evidence that the presence of social support, via marriage, frequent daily contact with others, or the presence of confidants, reduces mortality risk from cancer, as well as other diseases. In particular, expressive-social activities and social support, not merely being extraverted, have been found to be related to longer survival time (Hislop, Waxler et al., 1987; Waxler-Morrison, Hislop et al., 1991). These data confirm observations that emotional expression is associated with better medical outcome (Stavraky, Donner et al., 1988; Greer and Morris, 1975; Greer, Morris et al., 1979; Temoshok, 1985; Derogatis, Abeloff et al., 1979).

EFFECTS OF PSYCHOSOCIAL INTERVENTIONS ON HEALTH STATUS

Since social support and emotional expression have been shown to affect the rate of disease progression, structured psychotherapies designed to influence these factors might putatively have an effect on survival time. Providing social support interventions for isolated individuals under stress has been related to improved health outcome (Rodin, 1980, 1986; Raphael, 1977; Turner, 1981; Spiegel, Bloom et al., 1989; Richardson, Shelton et al., 1990; Fawzy, Kemeny et al., 1990; Fawzy, Fawzy et al., 1993; Forester, Kornfeld et al., 1985). There are comparatively few intervention studies testing this relationship between administered social support and survival time, but three of six randomized trials demonstrate such a relationship. In our group's randomized trial of supportive-expressive group therapy for women with metastatic breast cancer, there was a statistically significant eighteen-month average survival advantage for women in the group therapy condition at ten-year follow-up. Although there was no difference in median survival, by forty-eight months after the study had begun, all of the control patients had died and a third of the treatment patients were still alive (Spiegel, Bloom et al., 1989).

Data supporting this finding have emerged from two studies published since the original study. Richardson and colleagues (Richardson, Shelton et al., 1990), utilizing a randomized prospective design, found that a home visiting and educational intervention among lymphoma and leukemia patients resulted in longer survival time. Those patients who received the intervention were found to be more adherent to their medical treatment as measured by allopurinol usage. But even when this difference was controlled for statistically, intervention patients lived significantly longer than controls.

Similarly, Fawzy and colleagues (1993) found a survival advantage (3/40 vs. 10/40 deaths) at six-year follow-up for forty malignant melanoma patients randomly assigned to just six weeks of intensive group psychotherapy, compared with forty control patients. This UCLA group also observed significantly lower rates of recurrence (7/40 vs. 13/40) among the patients who had received group support. Recently, Dr. Fawzy informed us (personal communication) that these significant differences have continued at ten-year follow-up.

Four studies failed to find such a relationship. In two there were problems with the psychological intervention. Ilnyckyj and colleagues (1994) reported on a randomized intervention trial involving 127 cancer patients in several types of "supportive" group therapy, some professionally led, some patient directed. They observed no measurable psychological benefit of participation in the group programs compared to a routine care control condition, and also found no significant difference in survival time. An intervention that produces no improvement in psychological state is unlikely to influence survival time. This same problem is relevant to a more recent study by Cunningham and colleagues (1998). They attempted to combine educational and stress management techniques with a supportive-expressive intervention among metastatic breast cancer patients. They found no psychological or medical benefit, although outside of the randomized comparison, those patients who attended some kind of additional support group did live longer than those who did not. Gellert and colleagues (1993) compared subjects enrolled in the Exceptional Cancer Patient Program with a matched sample of cancer patients who had routine care. They found no difference in survival time between the two groups, confirming an earlier report from that group (Morgenstern, Gellert et al., 1984). This was a matching rather than a randomized trial examining a problematic intervention program (Spiegel, 1993b).

Linn and colleagues (1982) administered an individual psychotherapy program to a group of patients with carcinomas of the lung and gastrointestinal system. They found psychological benefit, but no effect on survival time in a well-conducted randomized trial. However, virtually all of the patients died during the first follow-up year. Thus it may be that the illness was so far advanced that it was too late for any possible psychosocial effect on disease progression. Also, these were different types of cancers from those examined in the other studies. It is possible, for example, that hormonal cancers such as breast cancer are more sensitive to psychosocial influences, although there were positive findings with malignant melanoma and lymphoma patients.

These studies provide evidence from three of six laboratories that conducted randomized trials that psychosocial intervention may increase survival time of cancer patients. In a review of the field of psycho-oncology, Greer called for further prospective studies and examination of biological mechanisms, stating that "the theoretical and practical implications of research in this area are considerable" (1993, p. 95)

CONCLUSION

It is clear from this research that the expression of relevant emotions and direct discussions of difficult subject matters enhances rather than hinders quality of life, and may actually increase survival time of women with breast cancer. The group experience offers to these patients a place in which they belong because of, rather than despite, their illness. Furthermore, it constitutes a place where they can express feelings that may upset them and their loved ones.

Fears about death and dying can be discussed openly, thereby helping to make thoughts about dying more tolerable. It provides emotional support, understanding, and validation of their experience. It can help members adjust to changes in their sense of self as well as their body image. There is an intense bonding among the members and a sense of acceptance through sharing a common dilemma. This serves to counter the social alienation that often divides cancer patients from their well-meaning but anxious family and friends.

Involvement in a group also allows patients to better mobilize their existing resources as well as develop new sources of support. Group members learn from one another, for instance, by modeling new and more effective means of coping with the illness. The interactive skills modeled and practiced in the group setting can be applied to other interactions as well. Techniques for improving the doctor–patient relationship and ultimately the medical management of their disease can be learned. Patients can become more effective partners in their own medical treatment. In addition, they can learn to clarify their needs from their family and friends and try out means of better meeting them. Thus group therapy provides an opportunity for obtaining mutual, family, social, and professional help.

Furthermore, group members come to feel better about themselves because they can use their experience with cancer to help others with the same disease. At a time when their resources seem to be diminishing, they can expand their domain of caring, support, and help to others. This makes them feel more engaged in life, even as their life is threatened and shortened by disease.

One area for future research involves the interaction between emotional expression and social support. Frequent and intimate social relationships both allow for and may encourage the expression of strong emotion. That, in turn, may stimulate the development of social support. This interaction is seen clearly in support groups for the medically ill, which can foster both.

Thus there is growing evidence that psychotherapy for the medically ill is a powerful and important treatment, with marked psychological and possible physical effects. We will be able to account for more variance in outcome and will be more effective in treating cancer patients as we advance our understanding of the role of psychotherapy in influencing both psychological and somatic coping with cancer.

PART TWO
STRUCTURING SUPPORT GROUPS FOR PATIENTS COPING WITH SERIOUS MEDICAL ILLNESS

CHAPTER 3

Guidelines for the Therapist in Structuring and Maintaining a Group

There are many issues to consider before beginning a supportive-expressive group for cancer patients. One of the first decisions is which patient population to target. Will you offer your group to patients with all types of cancer or focus on a single cancer population? Will you open your group to all stages of cancer or limit it to early or advanced stages? Will your group be time-limited and, if so, how long will it be? Will it be an open or closed group? Your answers to these questions will influence the type of group you assemble and are also likely to affect the types of issues that patients raise. Another consideration when beginning a group is ensuring that a safe and secure environment has been created. This includes addressing a number of issues at the outset, such as meeting with each new member prior to entering the group and making sure that appropriate group norms are established and inappropriate ones are discouraged. The group leaders' ability to convey empathy, genuineness, and to work in the here-and-now is also important for getting the group off to a constructive start. Each of these and related issues are described below.

CONSIDERING
TYPES OF CANCER

When deciding whether to include patients with all types of cancer or to focus on a single cancer, there are several considerations. From a strictly pragmatic viewpoint, you may find that a mixed group is preferable if you have a relatively small cancer population on which to draw.

A mixed cancer group may be composed of males and females. One advantage is that it is possible for members to deal directly with issues involving the opposite sex, such as concerns about whether he or she is still attractive to the opposite sex. However, it can also make it difficult to talk about such issues as sexual functioning. Your therapeutic skill will be important in modulating any inhibiting effects of a mixed group.

You will find that even though your members may have different cancers, they have many common concerns and experiences. Most of your patients will have endured, or will be undergoing, the physically and emotionally draining effects of radiation or chemotherapy. Most will be struggling with an altered self- and body image. Many will be concerned about the effect of the illness on their family and their relationships with others. Almost everyone will be fearful of dying from the disease. All of these shared concerns will serve to unify the group and build support and understanding. At the same time, however, it is important to be alert to concerns that are unique to each cancer patient.

One advantage to having a group for patients with all kinds of cancers is that it can sometimes broaden a patient's perspective on the illness and provide a greater sense of connection.

Paul, a young man with lung cancer, complained that he felt stigmatized because of the blame he felt others placed on him for getting cancer. "They don't even have to say it, you can just tell." Marjorie, a woman with breast cancer and herself a former therapist, relayed an experience she recently had in the parking lot. "I was sitting in my car and an old neighbor happened by and noticed me. She came over and stuck her head in my window and asked why I let myself get cancer. Intending to be helpful, she said to me, 'You caused your cancer; you can cure it.' I was so angry, I almost rolled the window up to strangle her. I realized later, after I calmed down," she chuckled, "that people who don't have cancer want to believe that we do it to ourselves because then they can reassure themselves that they are immune. So, Paul, I don't think this is so much about people blaming you for smoking. This is about people wanting to believe that they have control over their lives. The sad truth is that they don't. None of us do."

For Paul to hear that other cancer patients and not just lung cancer patients get blamed for their illness was important. If such a discussion took place in a group composed solely of lung cancer patients, it is much less likely that this kind of perspective would have been given.

Usually, however, we prefer to lead groups of patients with similar cancers, such as breast or prostate cancer. We find that there is an almost immediate sense of commonality among group members who have the same cancer. To some extent, however, this sense of shared understanding can be overinflated. A more realistic feeling of commonality tends to emerge over time as group members come to know each other and to understand their individual concerns. A statement that we hear time and again in these groups is the value patients feel from being with other people who know what they are going through.

Certainly, there are some kinds of encounters that we think would simply not occur in a mixed cancer group.

Mary had recently joined a breast cancer group after having been diagnosed with primary breast cancer. It had been several months since she'd had her mastectomy and she continued to struggle with her body—"damaged goods" as she put it. "I can't bear to look at myself in the mirror, let alone let anyone else see me. Who will ever love me with a body like this?" Several women began to encourage Mary to consider reconstructive surgery. Kristin listened quietly as the group members tried to convince Mary that she could reclaim her body through reconstruction. Following a moment of silence, Kristin turned to Mary and said, "Mary, I want to show you something," and she proceeded to unbutton her blouse to reveal her breast. "I had reconstructive surgery a year after my mastectomy because I also felt deformed and unlovable. I just wanted you to see what can be done. This is not the breast I had, but it is still my breast and it has allowed me to feel like a woman again. The funny thing is that while it has made a difference to how I feel about myself, having this breast or not having it has not seemed to matter to my husband one bit. He still loves me as much as he ever did. What it made me realize is that what matters is that I feel good about myself." Kristin buttoned up her blouse as the tears ran down Mary's face. This was a powerful moment for the group and a pivotal one for Mary.

It is unlikely such an encounter would have happened in a group that was not composed of women who shared the same illness.

CONSIDERING STAGE OF DISEASE

Whether to limit a group to certain stages of cancer is another important issue. We have found that including both primary and advanced cancer patients poses some difficulties, although it does have its advantages. From the point of view of the primary patients, one difficulty is that having individuals in the group with a more advanced stage of the disease can be frightening because it provides an all-too-graphic picture of what may be in store for them. It can be so frightening for some patients that it may result in their leaving the group. Most primary patients are clinging to the hope that the cancer has been cured. This can lead to a rejection of the advanced cancer patients by viewing them as different and in another category: "I'm not like her. That won't happen to me." The advanced cancer patient will already be struggling with a feeling of having been excluded from the mainstream. The rejection of the group members will only exacerbate this situation.

One of the problems that can emerge when limiting a group to patients with primary disease is that the disease may progress in one or more patients.

In one of our primary breast cancer groups, Melanie was diagnosed with metastatic disease. The progression of her disease threw both her and the group into crisis. One of her biggest fears was being ejected from the group and being left to die alone.

"I want to know whether it is okay with you if I stay in the group. I will have every understanding if it is not because the group is here for the majority, not the minority." There was a brief moment of stunned silence as the group members took in the devastating news. Doris, who was sitting beside Melanie, put her hand out to hold Melanie's hand and as the tears welled up in her eyes, said "Of course, I want to be with you through this." This sentiment was echoed by all the group members.

Although this particular group rallied around Melanie to support her, this is not always the case. We know of many instances when patients were left to feel that they no longer belonged after their disease progressed, which is a dangerous situation for all parties concerned.

Patients have been asked to leave because their disease progression makes them "bad" examples. However, our experience tells us that this is misguided. This is not only a terrible thing to do to the person whose cancer has progressed, implying that she is now unacceptable and somehow responsible for her misfortune, but it terrifies everyone else in the group—that is, there but for the grace of God go I. The fear of recurrence is universal. If patients are dismissed when they relapse, it gives the message that if you get sick, we will leave you, and if we're going to leave you, then maybe others will too. This is a central issue for all cancer patients—the fear of being abandoned and left to die alone. For the healthier patient, there is no guarantee that she will not be the next to have her disease progress. For the sick patient, she is in the throes of this fear and asking her to leave has made her fear a reality. Thus, regardless of the initial reactions of the group, we strongly urge you not to eject the member whose cancer has advanced.

Another potential difficulty for primary patients in a mixed-stage group is that patients with early-stage disease can feel that their concerns are trivial compared to those of the sicker members. However, we have found that this issue arises regardless of disease stage. In our metastatic groups, patients may have the same stage of disease but may be in different places in the disease process. For instance, some members might be dealing with active disease while others are experiencing a remission. Patients who are faring relatively well can feel that their concerns are not important enough to take up group time. We try to confront these issues head-on, usually by asking the worse-off group members whether they feel the other members' issues are trivial. Typically, the reply is a resounding "No!" with the added sentiment that everyone's concerns are important and they would hope that no one would ever think their own concerns were insignificant.

Even though problems may arise by having all stages of disease represented in the group, there is the potential for benefit. For the primary patients this comes from facing their worst fears. The fear of dying from cancer can be lessened by witnessing another person confront it. Primary patients can find that their fear is diminished by seeing the dreaded outcome before them. This concurs with our general approach to leading these groups, which is based on our belief that it is easier to cope with the worst fears if they are acknowledged and accepted. Seeing the acceptance of the metastatic patients and the support that is given can be tremendously reassuring. The metastatic patients often become role models and a source of inspiration on how to live in the face of dying.

> Esther responded to the concern of a patient with metastatic breast cancer that she was upsetting those who, like Esther, only had primary disease: "I used to think that if I ever got cancer, my life would be over. Well, I got cancer, and my life isn't over. Then I started thinking, if my cancer came back, my life would be over. Well, your cancer came back, and your life isn't over. Your being here helps me to understand that."

There are potential advantages for the metastatic patient as well. In facing a foreshortened future, there is usually a shift in priorities. Patients find themselves thinking carefully about what is important and meaningful for them given the time they have left. Being in a group with other people who are at earlier stages in the disease process gives the metastatic patients an opportunity to share the lessons they have learned about living with the illness. This can be a source of gratification for the metastatic patient and an inspiration for the patients with early-stage disease.

Even with the potential advantages of having all stages represented in a group, when given the choice, we prefer to have separate groups for our primary and advanced patients. Overall, we have found that the disadvantages outweigh the advantages. Even though both primary and advanced patients have issues and concerns in common, the potency and priorities in dealing with the issues differ when comparing the advanced and primary patients.

The main goal of many primary patients is to put the cancer behind them. In fact, this is often a problem because it can result in primary patients prematurely setting their fears aside. Sometimes primary patients think they are getting on with their lives and putting the cancer behind them, but actually they are trying to put their unresolved and uncomfortable fears and concerns out of their mind. Although this is often an issue for the primary patient, it is usually not an issue for the advanced patient, who is very much aware of having to live with the disease. These two orientations can sometimes lead to group members working at cross-purposes with each other. The advanced patients need to deal with their fear of death and the dying process, as well as completing their life tasks and any other unfinished business, mourning their losses, and making contingency plans for their care during the dying process—whereas, for many primary patients, these issues represent precisely the fears that they are trying to push out of their minds.

Marion was originally in one of our metastatic breast cancer groups but then moved out of the area and had to travel three hours to attend the group meetings. Because of the great distance she chose to attend our group once a month. Wanting a support group that she could attend on a more frequent basis, she joined a breast cancer support group in her community and found that she was the only woman with metastatic disease in the group. She attended that group for several months (while she also continued her monthly trek to our metastatic group) and eventually decided that her local breast cancer group was simply not meeting her needs. Surprisingly, what she told us was that in that group she found herself in the role of the caregiver as the women continually looked to her for information and advice. While she found this gratifying in the beginning, she eventually decided that she had other important needs that could only be met in a group with women who were in a similar situation.

Given these issues, we recommend that, whenever possible, you restrict your groups to either primary patients or advanced cancer patients in order to facilitate greater cohesion in your groups. We remind you, however, that in your primary cancer groups, one (or more) of your members may have their cancer spread or recur. If that happens, we urge you to work to keep the advanced cancer patient in your group. The members of your group will be frightened by this development and may want to make the problem disappear, but this will harm both the advanced cancer patient and the rest of the group. In time you may want to help your patient find an advanced cancer group. However, this should be done carefully and in a manner that does not communicate to your patient (or the group) that he or she no longer belongs.

OPTIMAL TIMING FOR
JOINING A GROUP

Another factor to consider is the timing of the group—that is, what is the optimal time for a patient to join a group? Should patients be advised to join a group as soon as they are diagnosed, during their medical treatment, or after they have completed their medical treatment? The psychiatric literature on crisis intervention (Caplan, 1964) suggests that there are certain times during the course of dealing with the disease that joining a group would be optimal. We have observed that the initial diagnosis and the period immediately after initial treatment ends are times of special stress (Fobair et al., 1986).

The distress caused by the diagnosis is obvious, but it is often mitigated by preoccupation with and hope for treatment procedures, coupled with supportive contact from health care personnel. The period after active treatment ends is surprisingly stressful, largely due to the withdrawal of frequent medical contact and support and the temporary cessation of active treatment. Treatment tends to counter both anxiety as well as cancer.

While there are many times of stress and potential benefit, we have observed that it is difficult to recruit patients to groups during the time immediately after diagnosis because patients and their families are so preoccupied with making treatment decisions and undertaking initial therapy. Indeed, in one study of an individual intervention, reduction in anxiety and depression was greater when patients received the intervention four months later rather than immediately after diagnosis (Edgar et al., 1992). We have found that for early-stage cancer patients, a group that bridges the time after treatment has been undertaken through the time after initial treatment ends seems effective. Providing group support during this period helps patients come to terms with the emotional aftereffects of the illness, which are particularly intense after medical treatment has been completed. For metastatic cancer patients, where the treatment course is ongoing and may be interspersed by periods of quiescence, the sooner patients get into a group and the longer they stay the better off they are.

THE LENGTH AND SIZE
OF THE GROUP

Depending upon the constraints of your work environment, you may or may not have much flexibility in deciding the length of your group. In terms of the optimal length of time, the research literature has reported benefits for groups as short as six or eight weeks (Cain et al., 1986; Fawzy et al., 1990a) and as long as twelve months (Spiegel et al., 1981, 1989). We have led groups for as short as twelve weeks (Classen, Koopman et al., in submission) and for as long as eight years (Classen, Butler et al., in submission). The optimal length of your group will depend upon your availability, resources, and the interest and needs of your patients.

In terms of patient need, we have found that advanced cancer patients derive significant benefit from a long-term group because their needs are chronic and extensive (Spiegel, Bloom, et al., 1981, 1989; Classen, Butler et al., in submission). For advanced patients we recommend at least a twelve-month intervention. In these groups, which usually involve individuals who will eventually die of their illness, continued participation in the group until death is valuable. We thus design these as ongoing groups, with new members added along the way. We have run such groups as long as eight years (and still going!). The ongoing sense of support through the process of dying and death is quite reassuring to members, and termination of such groups may rekindle anxiety about isolation and abandonment.

We have found that primary cancer patients can benefit from groups as brief as twelve weeks. Our research group is completing a study to demonstrate this benefit with primary breast cancer patients (Classen, Koopman et al., in submission; Spiegel, Morrow et al., 1996). Twelve weeks seems to be sufficient time to consolidate group cohesion and conduct the psychotherapeutic work. However, we have also learned that these women found the groups so beneficial that many of them continued to meet on their own after the twelve-week intervention, suggesting that even though a twelve-week intervention is helpful, perhaps more is better.

According to Yalom (1995), the optimal size for a psychotherapy group is between seven and eight members with an acceptable range of five to ten members. In almost any group you can expect one or two dropouts and this is no different in supportive-expressive cancer groups. Consequently, you may want to begin your group with nine to ten members. If you are leading an advanced cancer group, you may want to include as many as twelve members in your group because advanced cancer patients are much more ill and consequently more likely to be absent.

OPEN VERSUS CLOSED GROUPS

We have used closed groups for our brief (twelve-week) support groups, meaning that we did not allow new members to join after the first meeting. Our reason for closing these groups was to maximize the work that could be done in the allotted time. Allowing members to join your brief group a week or more after the group begins has two disadvantages. One is that it disrupts the group because you must shift your focus to introduce the group members to the new member and to establish a new cohesion in the group. Accomplishing this uses precious time. The second disadvantage is that the new member has even less time to benefit from the already brief support group.

For long-term groups we tend to have open groups where new members are permitted to join at any time, so long as there is still room in the group. An open group can be particularly important for long-term groups with advanced cancer patients. In advanced cancer groups you are likely to experience the death of group members or have members who are so gravely ill that they are unable to attend. An open group permits you to keep the group at an optimal size. This is important; one reason is that it can be very demoralizing for the surviving group members to have the group dwindle down to nothing. A caveat, however, is to be careful that you do not convey the message that you are replacing members. No one can be replaced. For this reason, we try to introduce new members to our groups in a way that is not contingent upon the loss of group members. Even so, you may find that the perception that you are replacing group members will need to be discussed.

PROVIDING A SAFE AND SUCCESSFUL
ENVIRONMENT FOR THE GROUP

The success of any group depends upon the environment that is created. Because the goal is to have members share their personal and intimate experiences, it is essential that the group be experienced as safe and consistent. Group members must know that at a given time each week the group will be there for them; that there is a predictability to the structure and function of the group; that what transpires in the group remains in the group; and that whatever they share about themselves is ultimately acceptable. Feeling free to share their experience does not mean that whatever they do, say, or feel will necessarily be liked or agreed with by the group. What is essential, however, is that each member know that he or she is acceptable *as a person* and that an individual can neither destroy nor be destroyed by the group.

In a cancer group where the goal is to support group members in their struggle to live with their disease, members must feel free to share their experiences and to respond honestly and openly to each other. Both sides of this equation—sharing and responding—are necessary if the group is to be a place where members feel supported in their efforts to live with cancer. Consequently, safety and consistency are important. In this section we discuss some general guidelines for ensuring that the groups you lead are experienced as safe and consistent. For a more in-depth discussion, see Irvin Yalom's seminal book on *The Theory and Practice of Group Psychotherapy* (Yalom, 1995).

CREATING AND SUSTAINING THE GROUP

Identifying Potential Members.   The group leaders are responsible for the creation and maintenance of the group. The first question to address in starting a group is, From where will you get your patients? Establishing a good working relationship with the radiation and oncology departments in your local hospital is a great place to start. Let them know who you are, including your credentials. You might tell them what kind of group or groups you are interested in conducting, what types of patients you are looking for, how long the group will last, and so on. Alternatively, you might inquire about what they see as the greatest need given their patient population.

Dr. James Roberts, a professor gynecological oncologist at Stanford University, approached us about our providing support groups for women with curable gynecological cancers. He felt that his patients had tremendous sexual and identity issues that emerged as a result of the horrendous surgeries many of them had to undergo. Instinctively, he knew they could not talk to him about these deeply personal concerns and he was searching for some other way to find them help with these issues. This suggests that it is worth getting to know the physicians who treat cancer patients and getting their perspective on which of their patients are in the greatest need of support groups. Working in concert with the treating physicians will increase the likelihood that you will service those patients who are in greatest need and that you will get maximum support from their physicians.

Payment.   Payment for such groups is usually not difficult, since the costs of one or two therapists' time and the use of facilties can usually be covered by relatively modest payments from each group member, usually on the order of one-fourth to one-fifth of the cost of individual psychotherapy. Some groups charge monthly fees, with the idea that each member makes a commitment to the others to attend regularly, and should pay for the space whether or not she can attend. More recently, however, the advent of managed care and HMO programs has restricted payment for groups, and many indemnity insurance programs do not cover supportive care.

Many patients and treatment programs have difficulty finding out what a given health plan covers. Some cover psychiatric care, but patients are reluctant to identify themselves as having a psychiatric problem in need of treatment. Also, there is growing competition in many communities from self-help or free support group programs, such as those provided by the Wellness Community. One way of dealing with these problems is to fund the group program from other sources, as some oncology treatment programs do. Clearly the complications of collecting the relatively modest fees needed to maintain a group therapy program underscore the need for better integration of group support into standard medical treatment.

Who Is Likely to Benefit?   Prior to starting a support group, it is helpful to identify the types of patients most likely to benefit. Of course, how to define *benefit* is a question all its own. While we do not have all the answers to this question, there are some recommendations and observations we can provide. In our study examining the benefits of a brief intervention for primary breast cancer patients, we discovered that it was only those women who were highly distressed who seemed to benefit from the support group when benefit was defined in terms of mood disturbance (Classen, Koopman et al., in submission). Thus, when we compared women who were randomly assigned to the twelve-week support group to women who were randomly assigned to the control group, it was those women who had the highest mood disturbance when they entered the study (approximately one-third of the sample) who showed the greatest improvement in mood disturbance over a two-year period. For those women who did not exhibit high initial mood disturbance, there was no measurable advantage to participation in group support: Both the treatment and control patients showed no change in mood disturbance over time. These results suggest that support groups should be offered to primary cancer patients who seem to be highly distressed about their disease.

Of course, there may be other ways to define *benefit*, and thus it is possible that it was not just the highly distressed patients who were helped in the groups. Those patients who were not highly distressed may have benefited from having the opportunity to share their experiences and concerns. The group may have enabled them to clarify their priorities or to teach them new coping strategies or to improve their communication with their families. Thus, these less distressed group members may have been helped in ways that we did not measure and therefore do not know.

Matching Patient Problems.   The success of your group will depend as much upon the group members as it does on what you bring to the group as the facilitator. Thus, adequate screening of potential group members is crucial in the creation of a group. When screening potential group members, it is useful to bear in mind the entire constellation of individuals you are bringing together. For instance, are there other group members with whom each person can identify? It is wise to have at least two people with a given major characteristic: having advanced disease, being married or single, being older, etc. Being an outlier in any group is often a setup for the person to become a scapegoat or to experience dissatisfaction.

> *Toni, a very masculine-appearing woman, was the only lesbian in a breast cancer group composed of white middle-class heterosexual women. When Toni came into the group, one of her first comments was to criticize the group leaders for not having more ethnic minorities in the group.*
>
> *We suspect that this was Toni's way of saying that she felt out of place and perhaps was looking for a reason to leave.*

> *To the group's credit, they tried very hard to welcome Toni. However, as hard as they and the group leaders tried to make Toni feel comfortable, she never did, and shortly thereafter left the group.*

Clearly, it was a mistake to bring her into this group where she had no other person with whom she could identify.

Patients with psychiatric problems should be assessed carefully for their appropriateness for group therapy. When an individual has difficulties that extend well beyond coping with cancer, both the individual and the group may be better served by having the person receive individual therapy in addition to or even instead of group therapy. In selecting group members, the aim is to include individuals who can both benefit from and contribute to the group experience.

Finding Members with Common Goals.   Another consideration is whether the goals of the potential member fit with the goals of the group as you see them. You can start by first asking the patient what he or she hopes to get out of joining a cancer support group. This provides an opportunity to learn about the patient's concerns, needs, and goals. It also provides the first indication of the compatibility of the patient's goals with the purpose of the group. It is important to learn the goals of the potential member to ensure that they do not conflict or compete with the overall goals of the group. For instance, if a potential group member is hoping to find a new set of friends with whom she can engage in social chitchat, this can seriously interfere with the purpose of the group.

Clearly stating the goals of the group as you see them can help the potential group member determine if his or her goals are compatible with those of the group. We had one member who stated that, because she was a longtime cancer survivor, her reason for being in the group was to provide hope for other members. What she did not state was that she was in a crisis in her life because she was in the middle of a divorce. Her unstated goal was to have a place where she could vent and be supported during this process. This patient's unstated goal served to derail the group from its purpose, which was, of course, to focus on cancer. After several months of struggle on both her part and that of the group, she opted to leave. This situation could have been avoided had we carefully examined at the outset her stated goal of wanting to be a "beacon of hope." Implicit in this goal was that she did not feel the need for support in relation to her cancer. Both she and the group would have benefited had we identified her real needs at the outset.

The purpose of the group experience should be discussed with prospective members. Because there is a natural resistance to talking about such frightening topics as death and dying, it can be helpful to address this issue at the outset. Many patients have adopted the unfortunate but prevailing view in our society that positive thinking is essential for either preventing or curing cancer. This has been interpreted to mean that cancer patients should avoid thinking about any negative topics such as the possibility that the cancer may recur and possibly lead to death. There are two problems with this view. One is that it puts a tremendous burden on cancer patients and, in effect, holds them responsible for their cancer. The other is that concerns about the cancer and fears of dying exist whether people decide to talk about them or not. Our belief is that it is actually more positive to talk about these concerns than to expend a lot of energy trying to repress them. We believe that, by talking about their fears, patients will learn better ways of coping with them and ultimately defuse them of much of their power. This rationale should be stated clearly to all prospective members.

There are many ways to describe the basic philosophical approach to leading these groups. The following is one example of introducing the purpose of the group at the initial group meeting:

Before we begin I'd like to to say a few words about the purpose of this group. When most people learn they have cancer, they typically have two types of reactions. One reaction, as was aptly described by one of you, is "shock and terror." In fact, often the first thing that comes to mind is the fear that you're going to die. The second reaction is that you can feel terribly alone because no one seems to understand what is happening to you. What we hope to do in our group is to provide a place where you can talk about all the things that concern you about having cancer—including the scary stuff like, "What if this disease kills me?"—as well as providing a place where you will feel supported and less alone. Our main purpose is to help each of you cope with this disease. My role as the group leader will be to help you to share your experiences and to support each other. My hope is that you will find that this group is a place where you feel safe and free to talk about any concerns you might have about living with this disease.

If your group is part of a research study, it is important to remind the members of that fact. No doubt, there will be questionnaires to complete and/or additional interviews to be scheduled. The purpose of the study should be clearly stated and, of course, written informed consent obtained.

Members with Additional Problems. During the screening process it is also a good idea to be alert to any foreseeable problems so that you can try to prevent them from developing. Although problems can emerge in many forms, there are some common issues to which you should be alert. Sometimes by identifying the issues that might make it difficult for the member to participate fully, it is possible to lessen their effect. For example, for patients who have other major life issues with which they are also struggling, it is helpful to discuss what they are doing to deal with these issues and how comfortable they will feel focusing on cancer-related issues. At this time it might even be appropriate to recommend additional therapy so that patients have a place to work on their other problems. This can go a long way toward keeping your group from being sidetracked.

If the patient states that she believes it is important to think positively, it is crucial that you address this issue at the outset because this patient's orientation may be at odds with the goals of the group. Ask your patient what she means by thinking positively. Does your patient find it helpful to talk about her fears, such as the fear of dying from the disease? If so, does this mean that she is not being positive?

After hearing your patient's perspective, you can then provide your own. You might find that there is very little disagreement between the two of you, or that there is resistance to your approach. This topic often requires a lot of attention because many patients find it uncomfortable to talk about difficult issues and truly believe that it is physically detrimental to have "negative" feelings. Beginning this discussion prior to the group's commencement will likely make your patient more open to the issue when it arises in group.

Establishing Boundaries. When you are interviewing potential patients, it is important to state the basic structure and time frame of the group. The aim here is to establish the boundaries of the group. You should say when, where, and for how long the group will be held. Respecting the confidentiality of group members should be discussed. Unlike most psychotherapy groups, we encourage members to contact each other outside of group if they desire. This

is in keeping with one of the main goals of the group, which is to enhance social support and is different from merely widening one's circle of friends.
Friendships may develop, but the support is focused on coping with cancer
together.

It is also a good idea to talk about group maintenance issues, such as the
importance of regular attendance, arriving on time, and members informing
the leaders in advance if they are going to be absent. Arriving on time and
regular attendance are desirable both for the individual and for the group.
Obviously, arriving late is disruptive to the group, but it also diminishes
what the tardy member can get from the group. While it is important in any
group to address issues of member absences, it is particularly important in
cancer groups. Not commenting upon and inquiring into absences can lead
to an underlying fear among the group that each of them can slip away unnoticed. In cancer groups an absence can generate deep concern and anxiety
about the absent member's health. It is important for these reasons that any
absence be followed up by the leader before the next group meeting and that
the group be informed at the next meeting about the reason for the absence.

Thoroughly preparing your prospective group members should set the
stage for a productive and cohesive group. It will enable you to begin forming a good working alliance, to ensure that each member is suitable for the
group, and to deal with any issues that might have the potential of disrupting the group's work. The group members must understand the nature of the
group in which they have agreed to participate. This will work against competing expectations developing and potentially disrupting the group process.

SHOWING EMPATHY AND
UNCONDITIONAL POSITIVE REGARD

Carl Rogers (1957) considered empathy, unconditional positive regard, and
genuineness as "necessary and sufficient conditions" for therapeutic change.
We take the position that these conditions are necessary, although not sufficient, for reaching our goals in supportive-expressive group therapy.

Empathy is the cornerstone of any psychotherapeutic approach. It involves having an accurate understanding of the patient point of view and
experiencing it as if it were your own. It is important to emphasize that it is
as if the patient's experience were your own. Maintaining this stance ensures
that the therapist does not get lost in the patient's experience or confuse his

or her own experience with that of the patient. An empathic reflection does not require that the therapist repeat back to the patient everything that has been said. Instead, it often involves sidestepping much of what has been said in order to reflect the underlying meaning (Rogers, 1970). An empathic response conveys to the group member a sense of being understood and accepted and that one is not alone.

A therapist has unconditional positive regard for a group member if he or she feels a warm acceptance of all aspects of the person's experience. Unconditional positive regard does not mean that the therapist necessarily approves of everything the patient says or does. Nevertheless, there is a sincere respect for the patient as a separate and valuable person. Both empathy and unconditional positive regard are essential for providing an environment of safety, enabling the group members to lay bare their fears and anxieties about living with cancer. One particularly poignant example of the power of empathy occurred in one of our metastatic breast cancer groups.

Sarah was a gentle, reserved, and soft-spoken 70-year-old woman who for the past several months had become increasingly ill. She came into group one day distraught because of an encounter she had had with one of her doctors. She had wanted to get some information from him about the state of her illness and was frustrated because she could not find out what she wanted. Sarah was clearly upset as she talked about this situation and her concern about her health. The group members, who loved her dearly, rallied around her to support her efforts to get the information she wanted from her doctor. They suggested numerous things she might say or things she might do, to the point that it felt as though she was being barraged with well-intentioned but ultimately unsatisfying advice.

As the group leader listened and watched, she was struck by the series of emotions that passed over Sarah's face. Finally the leader interrupted the conversation and said, "Sarah, it is really clear to me that everyone in this group wants more than anything to help you. Yet, I've noticed that while people have been giving you all these suggestions you've had a lot of different reactions and I'm sensing that we are not giving you what you need right now." Sarah got choked up as she began to talk: "I just want to know because my family is going to be coming home for Christmas and . . ." The group leader thought she understood what Sarah was too afraid to say and gently probed, "Sarah, are you afraid you are going to die before you see them?" The shift that occurred because of this empathic response was remarkable. Sarah, who was usually self-contained, broke down sobbing as she finally communicated what was on her mind. The response of the

group was to shower her with love and support and Sarah, for the first time, was able to
speak about her deepest fears.

As much as the group leaders strive to maintain an empathic and accepting stance in relation to the group members, ruptures in the therapeutic relationship are bound to occur from time to time. Ruptures occur when a member feels that the therapist does not understand or accept her experience. The experience of the rupture may or may not be due to actual empathic failure on the part of the group leader. Sometimes it is due to the misperception of the member. On the other hand, it may very well be due to the leader's lack of empathic understanding. Whatever the real cause of the rupture, it is essential that the therapist seek to mend the break.

Such a situation occurred in one of our groups. Unfortunately, the rupture was not apparent to the group leaders and it was not until several months later that the member was able to address it. The incident occurred early on in the life of the group when the patient was describing a difficult situation. While describing this situation to the leader, she incorrectly stated the leader's name, to which the leader responded by correcting her. What the patient was unable to say was that she perceived the leader as caring more about being named correctly than about the patient's concerns. This was experienced as an empathic failure. In time the patient came to feel again the leader's empathy and caring for her and eventually was able to speak about the incident with her. This example speaks to the need for group leaders to be on guard for situations that might be experienced as empathic failures.

SHOWING GENUINENESS

Rogers describes showing genuineness as being congruent with your own internal experience (1957), also referred to by Yalom as "transparency" (1995). Being congruent with your internal experience requires self-awareness—a prerequisite for any therapist. In the context of working with cancer patients, group leaders should be aware of the countertransference issues that this subject evokes. It is necessary for group leaders to recognize if and when their internal reactions to what is unfolding in group has the potential to affect the group negatively. There are several issues that are commonly evoked by working with cancer patients and there are likely to be other issues that are unique to the therapist. The group leaders have a responsibility to examine themselves and to be alert to the potential their countertransference has to impede the group work.

One issue that is bound to arise as we work with cancer patients is confronting our own mortality. Although we all know intellectually that we are destined to die, it is another matter to face this realization emotionally. As difficult as it may be, you should try to be aware of the feelings that emerge for you when this topic comes up. This is such a frightening topic for many of us that it is not unusual to find it difficult to access any feelings about the subject. Even if a numbing of your emotional response is all that you are aware of, it is important to recognize that this is what you are feeling. If this is your response to the subject and you are not aware of it, it is possible that you will seek to avoid this topic and have no awareness that you are doing so. Often simply being aware of one's feelings is sufficient to keep one's own reaction from impeding the group work.

Many therapists who lead cancer support groups have had a personal brush with the illness. Some are themselves cancer survivors. Others may see themselves as being at risk for the disease because of a family history or have had occasion to worry that they had the disease. Still others may have had the experience of having had someone they care about develop cancer or, worse still, have lost someone to cancer. Each of these experiences has the potential to raise significant countertransference issues for the group leader.

Memories and feelings about past losses, regardless of the cause of death, can be triggered when one leads a cancer support group. Facing the possibility of a member's death or an actual death can activate feelings about other losses. Sometimes it can be difficult to tell whether the sadness is solely in response to the group. At other times it may be clear to the leader that he or she is reexperiencing a personal loss. In either case, it is important for the leader to recognize his or her own internal response. Most losses we experience in the course of our lives tend to reevoke earlier losses. What is important is that we recognize when our feelings are too much or too strong to be in response to the group. If this occurs it is usually an indication that the leader has some private grief work to do.

Fear is another reaction that can be experienced when leading a cancer support group. No one is immune to developing cancer, and when you lead a cancer support group this fact is hard to deny or ignore. The effect of this recognition seems to be especially acute with leaders who are new to the field. We have talked to novice group leaders who find themselves so gripped by this fear that they seriously question whether they are cut out to do this work. In most cases, these therapists have found enormous relief by talking about the fears and concerns, in conjunction with learning that these reactions are not unusual, but instead are a natural response. Nevertheless, the occasional therapist may decide that this is an area in which he or she is unprepared or unwilling to work. These therapists are to be commended for their self-awareness and integrity.

Identification with particular group members can intensify a group leader's countertransference. Similarities in gender, age, profession, life stage, medical history, or other characteristics can result in identification or even overidentification with the patient. The result can be healthy mirroring of the patient's emotions by the group leader. Alternatively, the leader may run the risk of losing his or her therapeutic perspective if the leader over-identifies. In such a situation, the therapist is likely to require consultation with an experienced clinician for help in reestablishing boundaries. Ordinarily, it is relatively easy for therapists to recognize the individuals with whom they most identify. Acknowledging this identification within yourself, as well as sharing it with your co-leader, is important. This will enable both you and your co-leader to be alert for any potential countertransferential problems that might arise.

As in any therapy, it is mandatory that therapists be aware of the ways in which they are affected by the therapeutic process. In some respects, leading cancer support groups can be unusually challenging. It is difficult to watch patients struggle with something about which neither they nor we have any control. They feel helpless and we too can feel the same. This is unlike other forms of therapy where we, as therapists, often feel that there is something we can do. With cancer groups often the best we can do is simply *be* there.

There are many ways in which you can be affected by leading a cancer support group. In this regard, your primary goal should be to become conscious of the ways in which the group is affecting you. Second, you need to decide what to do about it. There are several options. One is simply to acknowledge it to yourself. Another is to seek outside consultation if your reaction feels too intense and intrusive to the group process. The third option is to share your response with the group.

By becoming aware of your own internal experience, you can then decide the extent to which it is appropriate to share the experience with the group. Usually it is not so important or necessarily helpful that the therapist share his or her internal experience with the group, but it is essential that you be aware of it. One of the issues to consider here is genuineness. To be genuine requires that your internal response be congruent with what you are communicating. To be congruent or genuine, Rogers (1961) believed that the feelings the therapist is experiencing should be available to his or her awareness and that the therapist be able "to live these feelings, be them, and able to communicate them if appropriate" (Rogers, 1961, p. 61). This suggests that genuineness does not require communicating what one is feeling but it does require that we know what our feelings are and that the way we are is not discrepant with them.

There are times when self-disclosure can be beneficial to the group. Yalom (1995) considers "therapist transparency" as a potentially powerful tool in group therapy. However, he cautions that it be used judiciously. The needs of all the group members must be taken into consideration because what may be beneficial for some group members may not be beneficial for all. The ultimate principle in making decisions about self-disclosure is not honesty, but responsibility. When making a decision to self-disclose, the therapist must be clear how this will benefit and not hinder the group. Self-disclosure can function as a model for the group.

Marilyn consistently arrived late to group and when she did she would usually be disruptive by somehow calling attention to herself. Today was no exception. She arrived at group in the middle of an important discussion of loss. Because she had been confronted about her disrupting the group in the past, she waited ten minutes before speaking during a pause in the discussion. She said, "Where's Rebecca?" After being given what information there was about Rebecca, she said, "I'm sorry I'm late but I lost track of the time because of a letter I received in the mail today from my friend who has AIDS. It is a really powerful letter that I would like to read to the group. I think it is really relevant to what we all deal with. Would you like me to read it?" As she looked around the group for members' permission, one of the leaders sighed and then spoke up. "Marilyn," he said, "I don't know how to bring this up easily, but I find myself feeling annoyed because you are late and it makes it hard for me to want to listen to you read the letter." Marilyn replied, "I'm sorry I was late but I waited ten minutes before I spoke so that I wouldn't interrupt things." The leader responded, "It's true you did, but I still find it disruptive." Marilyn stated, "Well, you and I have gone over this before. I think this is old material and I don't want to waste any more of the group's time on it." "Well, perhaps it's just me. But I think we should hear what other people think," he replied. Marilyn reluctantly agreed and they turned to the group members for their reaction.

This led to each of the group members, without exception, talking about the ways in which they found it disconcerting to have Marilyn arrive late. Some people were annoyed and others worried about her when she wasn't there. Everyone agreed that it was always disruptive.

This was a difficult but important discussion that enabled the group members to air thoughts and feelings they had been harboring for some time. Surely it would not have occurred had the group leader not had the courage to speak genuinely about his annoyance.

Self-disclosure can be particularly effective if the therapist has personally faced a life-threatening disease. If the leader has had cancer, self-disclosure can serve many purposes. One of the most powerful effects is that it may function as a source of hope. Knowing that the therapist underwent the same experience, was able to work it through, and go on with her life can be tremendously encouraging. It can also enhance the patient's sense of feeling understood and less alone and can give patients courage to face many of the frightening issues that cancer raises.

However, most leaders have not had the experience of facing a life-threatening disease. In spite of this, we all share the reality of an uncertain future. Death can just as easily claim a group leader as a group member. While it is true that healthy individuals do not live with the continual threat of having the sword of Damocles hanging over their head, as one of our patients liked to describe it, their future is just as uncertain. Consequently, as you lead these groups and as you pay attention to your internal process, you may notice your own anxieties and fears lingering beneath the surface. Sharing this internal experience in an appropriate fashion can sometimes help to lessen the sense of isolation that patients often feel when they are with people who are healthy.

Establishing Group Norms

An essential component in beginning any group is establishing group norms, otherwise known as "culture building" (Yalom, 1995). Group norms are the set of implicit or explicit behavioral rules by which a group conducts itself. These behavioral rules can be stated explicitly by the group leaders, although often they are imparted through role modeling. Group norms can also be introduced implicitly by the members and it is the job of the leaders to ensure that such behavioral rules are in the interest of the group.

The role of the therapist is to facilitate the establishment of a set of norms that, at their most basic level, will contribute to an environment of safety and acceptance. Conditions of safety and acceptance serve as a foundation from which the group can work. In order for the group to engage in the work of group therapy, there are a number of additional norms that must be established. Members must feel free to interact spontaneously and honestly with each other. This is especially important in a supportive-expressive therapy group since one of the active ingredients in this therapy is the support that members give to each other.

Spontaneity.   When a group first begins, there is a tendency for group members to take turns speaking. This is a norm you will quickly want to discourage. In virtually every cancer group we have observed, the initial meeting consists of the group members going around the room and describing their cancer history. In terms of norms, there are two issues here: One has to do with *how* the members are participating and the second has to do with *what* they are communicating. The *how* refers to the tendency for one member to speak uninterruptedly as she tells her personal story, followed by the person next to her, and so on around the room. Thus, rather than a spontaneous interaction among group members, there is a rigid and formal means of communication. The *what* refers to the tendency for cancer patients to describe the "facts" about their cancer experience with little or no reference to their emotional response to these events. The group leaders can work against the development of these norms during the first session by asking about the patient's feelings as he or she relays his or her "story" or about the emotional responses of others as they listen.

In early groups there is a tendency to look to the group leaders for direction. Often members will speak directly to the leaders rather than to each other. This is something to be discouraged. One effective way of discouraging a dependence upon the leaders for answers or direction is to seize any opportunity that arises to redirect questions asked of the group leaders to the group—for example, "I'm wondering if the group has any thoughts about your question?"

Authentic, spontaneous, and supportive interaction among group members is a central norm to establish. Sometimes it may not appear possible for a group member to be both authentic and supportive with another group member. This occurs, for example, when members are in disagreement or conflict with each other. Perhaps the most critical issue here is that members and leaders have a nonjudgmental acceptance of each other. Differences must be tolerated. In this regard the therapist may need to intervene occasionally to protect a group member or to facilitate a dialogue between members who are in conflict. If underlying tensions exist, it is important to work them through sufficiently so that they do not create an unsafe working environment.

Acceptance of Religious Differences.   One area in which you may find differences among group members is religious orientation. This topic is likely to arise in cancer groups given the life-threatening situation of the group members. In one of our breast cancer groups religious faith has frequently come up as a topic. We have some members with a very strong Christian faith and others who are avowed atheists. In spite of the profound differences in their beliefs, these women have learned to hear and respect each other's point of view. It is not a topic that they go out of their way to avoid, nor is it one that they dwell on. Each of these women has developed a genuine respect and acceptance of the others.

Open Discussion of Conflict.   When conflict does arise among group members, it can be a challenging issue to manage. The best-case scenario is when the group members are willing to talk through their disagreement in an attempt to understand each other's perspective. The worst cases are when group members express their feelings but are unwilling to engage in a dialogue or, worse still, do not express their feelings at all but keep them brewing inside. We have had the experience of discovering long after the fact that a member has been upset with another member or perhaps a group leader and had decided not to bring it up in group.

> *Sally was so angry at another member, Charlotte, that she seriously considered leaving the group. It wasn't until Charlotte died many months later that Sally finally told the group about her feelings. Although it was fortunate that Sally dealt with it sufficiently within herself that she was able to continue coming to group, it was not the optimal situation. Both she and Charlotte were denied the opportunity of working it out between them. The rest of the group was deprived of the opportunity to learn from Sally and Charlotte confronting each other honestly and finding a means of resolution.*

When these kinds of events happen, it is important to consider whether there is something about the group culture that prevents group members from speaking about these difficult issues.

Self-Disclosure. Self-disclosure is another important norm to be established in groups. Many argue that it is the most important norm because without self-disclosure there would be no material to work with in the groups and, ultimately, no benefit. The issue of self-disclosure is complex, however. As Yalom (1995) explains, self-disclosure is a subjective phenomenon and therefore difficult to assess objectively. What is extremely self-revealing for one person may not be for another. Thus, it is the subjective assessment of self-disclosure that is critical. The most important aspect of self-disclosure, according to Yalom, is that it is an interpersonal act. He believes that what is self-disclosed is less important than the fact that it is told to others. Consequently, when there is self-disclosure it is important to explore the person's thoughts and feelings around the disclosure as well as the reactions of others.

Related to the issue of self-disclosure is group participation at a more general level. Although all members are expected to participate in discussions, it is not unusual to find that some members are much more active than others. The role of the therapist is to be sure that there is room for everyone to participate. Sometimes this involves sensitively managing a patient who tends to leave little room for others to participate. At other times, with silent or near silent members, the therapist may need to encourage members to voice their thoughts and feelings. Even with consistent and thoughtful interventions, you may find that some individuals continue to speak very little while others tend to dominate. This is an indication that you must continue to play an active role in helping each group member find a way to be an active participant.

INITIAL SESSION

The first session of therapy is important because it sets the stage for what is to come. In supportive-expressive cancer groups there are several objectives that should be accomplished in the first meeting: (1) providing a rationale to the members regarding the aims of the group and how it will proceed; (2) introducing members to each other; and (3) identifying the expectations and goals of each member. There is an additional objective, which is not stated to the group: beginning the development of the group culture.

STATING GROUP RULES AND GOALS

In providing a rationale to the group, a number of issues should be addressed. Although most of this information will have been provided in screening and preparatory sessions, it is helpful to repeat it. Thus, you can remind the members that the purpose of the group is to provide a place where they can deal with the impact of the cancer on their lives. They are invited and encouraged to raise all issues, concerns, thoughts, and feelings that they have about any aspect of this disease and its consequences for them. Hopefully, they will find the group to be a place where they feel safe and supported. Your role as group leaders is to facilitate and support each member in this endeavor.

Along with stating the purpose and goals of the group, it is important to remind the members of the structure of the group and rules regarding confidentiality and attendance. If your group is time limited, you will want to remind them of the number of sessions. If it is an open group, you should state this as well as your policy about admitting new members to the group. Do you plan to inform the members ahead of time when a new person will be joining the group? This is always a good idea. Do you plan on including the group in the decision about whether or not there is room for another member? Clearly these are issues that you should resolve ahead of time.

Encourage members to attend regularly and whenever possible to inform the group about anticipated absences or, at the very least, to phone the group leaders before the session. Although this is important in any group, in a cancer support group absences take on special meaning because of the natural concern for each other's physical well-being. In general, we recommend that you begin each meeting by taking stock of who is present and to account for any absences. Unexplained absences can raise several questions for the group members. Is something wrong? Has the member taken a turn for the worse? Will people care if I am absent? Would people notice? These questions and others can be brewing beneath the surface if you are not careful.

Confidentiality should be given special attention and a consensus should be reached. The usual stance regarding confidentiality in group therapy is that what is spoken about in group remains in group. However, a cancer support group is not a psychotherapy group and therefore the issues are somewhat different. For instance, unlike psychotherapy groups, we encourage the group members to have contact with each other outside of group. Consequently, find out from your group members what level of confidentiality feels comfortable. Is it acceptable to speak to their spouses about what transpires in group? Is it okay to identify who is in the group? Is it acceptable to speak about some issues (such as a member's health status) but not others (such as sexual problems)? This discussion is critical for creating an atmosphere of trust. Because of its importance, and especially if you plan to introduce new members to the group in the future, you may need to revisit the issue again down the road.

INTRODUCTIONS

The first session is the time to ask the members to introduce themselves to each other. As way of introduction ask them to state who they are, to provide a brief history of their disease, and what they hope to get out of the group. These introductions generally take up most of the first session and sometimes it is necessary to complete the introductions in the second session. It is clearly preferable to complete the introductions in the first meeting. One way to ensure this is, prior to the first introduction, to remind the group how much time is left and ask everyone to keep that in mind so that there is time to complete introductions.

During the course of introductions, it is not unusual for members to introduce emotionally difficult material. This is a productive beginning to any group. However, it requires special attention. It is important to be supportive and, if possible, to facilitate some exploration. But, unlike the meetings that follow, topics that are introduced during this first session should not be allowed to dictate the course of the entire first meeting. For a leader, the issues to keep in mind are to be sure that people feel supported if they bring up difficult material and that there be enough time for everyone to speak. Thus, it is preferable to have all members introduce themselves before the group charges forward. Once this is accomplished, and if time allows, then it is a good idea to return to any important topics that have been introduced.

SUMMARIZING IMPORTANT THEMES

Following the introductions it can be helpful to summarize what you have heard. The aim is to summarize in terms of the themes that have emerged. This presents the first opportunity to reinforce the topics that you believe are important in a group of this nature. Thus, you might summarize by stating that some of the issues that most of them seem to be struggling with include their fear of dying from this disease, adjusting to a new image of self and body, and so on. You may find that there are some issues that were not mentioned. This may be because these issues do not concern them or possibly that they were too difficult to broach. Consequently, it can be helpful to mention these issues as additional topics that they may or may not want to discuss in the future.

The initial session is unique in that you will come with an agenda for the group. Although we encourage you to try your best to accomplish the objectives we have outlined, don't worry if you find that you have run out of time. Whatever remains can easily be addressed in the following session.

EARLY SESSIONS

In this section we describe strategies to keep in mind in the early sessions of your group. These strategies are also described in greater detail in later chapters. Your main goals in the early stages of the group are twofold: to establish a safe working environment and to facilitate the development of the group culture. Essentially, your aim should be to create an environment where the group members feel safe enough to talk about all aspects of their experience in living with cancer. In addition, you should facilitate development of a group culture where emphasis is placed on the expression of thoughts and feelings about living with the disease and on supporting each other.

We adopt five general strategies to accomplish these goals in the early sessions. One is to allow the group process to unfold in as natural a way as possible. In other words, we want to allow the group members to interact in ways that will enable them to feel comfortable in the group. A second is that we seize opportunities to access the feelings underlying the discussion. Third, we gradually move toward facilitating active coping strategies. A fourth strategy is to facilitate group interaction so that members will feel included and will begin to form supportive relationships with each other. Finally, we work to keep the focus on cancer.

ALLOW TOPICS TO EMERGE NATURALLY

There are likely to be specific things that each individual needs to do in order to feel comfortable sharing his or her life with a group of strangers. At the beginning this usually involves telling their stories. Consequently, and as mentioned earlier, this is something that we build into the structure of the first meeting. Following the first meeting, however, we provide much less structure. That is, we allow the group to determine the focus of the meeting.

In the early sessions especially, you will find that your members will talk about their medical treatment, including treatment regimens and their experiences with the medical profession. This is to be expected given that this is one topic about which everyone identifies and about which it is easy to talk. Thus, it can provide a means by which people get to know each other and thereby begin to develop feelings of safety and trust in the group. Notwithstanding the benefits of these discussions, this topic is a tricky one because it can also serve as a way of avoiding more difficult issues. Consequently, in the early meetings you might allow these discussions to take their natural course. However, over time you should begin to listen carefully for any emotions that may be hovering beneath the surface. Having to deal with chemotherapy, radiation, surgery, side effects of treatment, plus endless doctor's appointments, and sometimes less than satisfactory relationships with one's physician can raise difficult feelings and concerns. Helping the group members to work through these experiences is important.

Although discussions about treatment can present opportunities to explore members' affective responses to treatment, these topics can also keep the group from dealing with more difficult issues. It is easy for a cancer support group to function such that members talk at an informational level about their medical treatment, for instance by comparing their treatment regimens or talking about the newest available treatment. Often the group members find that this is genuinely helpful. They might learn about new treatments that they can pursue with their doctors or they might receive helpful information about what side effects to expect and how to deal with them. Because these benefits are real and there is usually a strong desire to have these sorts of discussion, it is important to allow them to take place. However, be aware that these discussions are also a potential trap.

Sometimes discussions about treatment are a way of dealing with anxiety about the disease, and particularly in the early stages of the group, they can even be a way of dealing with anxiety about being in a support group. Consequently, you should always be alert to the possibility that these kinds of discussions are occurring in order to avoid more difficult issues.

Encourage Exploration of Emotion

As your group matures, you will find that less and less time is spent on superficial topics. This is because you will have been shaping the culture in such a way that the group knows that they are there to focus on deeper issues. How will you do that? One rule of thumb we recommend is that, from the moment the group starts, you should be alert to affect. In fact, if there were only one recommendation we could give you, it would be to focus on the affect in the room. This orientation is one that you should rely on throughout the life of your group.

There are many ways in which affect can be expressed. You can recognize affect by the crack in the voice while a person is speaking, by the sudden break in speech as the person attempts to regain composure, by the unusual choice or emphasis of a word, by the sudden shift in topic, or by tears welling in the person's eyes. These nonverbal cues are telling you that there are some strong feelings beneath the surface. When you observe any of these cues, shift your focus immediately to the behavior that indicated affect. Often this will mean interrupting the person. It can be as simple as saying, "It looks as if that stirred up some feelings. Can you tell us about them?" or "What came up for you just now?" We recommend that you interrupt rather than wait for a natural opening. By waiting you often lose the affect and instead get an intellectualized explanation. As you learn to listen for affect, you will find that affect guides you toward the most important material. We recommend adopting this strategy in the early sessions so that you can immediately begin developing the desired culture.

When you notice an emotional reaction in a member who is not speaking, we suggest a slightly different strategy. Such is the case when someone starts to cry while another is speaking. In these situations, it is usually more appropriate to wait for the speaker to complete his or her thought before shifting the focus to the crying member. However, as in all situations, you will need to use your clinical judgment regarding the right time to shift the focus from the speaker to the other member. If the speaker is discussing something of great importance to him or her, you may need to wait a significant length of time before you turn to someone else.

When you are successful in shifting the focus to the affect, you are likely to find that there is an immediate deepening in the discussion, often leading directly to the heart of the matter for this individual. This usually has an effect on the other members as they tend to match the level of the discussion. In fact, when this doesn't happen, you should pay close attention. The members who shift to a more superficial level may be struggling with their emotional reaction to the discussion. It might also reflect that the group is in the early stages of development.

WHEN TO FACILITATE ACTIVE COPING

Although you should gradually move toward the facilitation of active coping strategies, we caution you not to move there too soon. As a group leader you may find it difficult to listen to your group members' fears and pain and consequently you will feel a strong desire to help solve their problems. As a result, you may run the risk of prematurely jumping in to help your patients feel better. Thus, we urge you to proceed cautiously. If you are in doubt as to whether it is the appropriate time to shift the focus to coping, ask yourself "Am I wanting to shift the focus to coping because I am feeling uncomfortable with the feelings that this brings up in me?" If you sense that you are doing it to make yourself feel better, you are advised to wait. Instead, you might want to use your own internal reaction as a way to express empathy for the patient or to encourage others to share their responses to what they have heard.

Before shifting the focus to coping strategies, it is important that the problem the person is struggling with has been adequately explored. If this has not occurred, then you or the patient may not fully understand the nature of the problem. As a result, you are unlikely to come up with a coping strategy that truly addresses the problem. For the same reason, you should be alert to when the group members rush in to offer solutions to a member in distress.

> *Meredith came to a meeting in a state of extreme distress and despair. She talked about things "disintegrating" around her, particularly involving people who were closest to her. It turns out that Meredith had introduced a female friend of hers to her partner of five years, and that he and her friend had been spending a lot of time together and had gotten very close. He recently decided to discuss his "feelings" for the friend with Meredith. Meredith was feeling especially vulnerable and felt this was the wrong time for him to be giving her such information. She described being angry and upset. In the process she also referred to herself as "the cancer person." One of the co-leaders asked what she meant by that and Meredith started to reel off the list of things that have happened to her as a result of her diagnosis. She lost her job, is living on disability, she has an 85 percent chance of recurrence, Don is afraid of losing her and he now has her friend there to console him. To this, one of the members immediately responded that Meredith should "dump" Don. Another member jumped in to agree.*

The therapists need to intervene in this type of situation. It is premature to be talking about what coping strategy to use to deal with Don. Instead, the focus should turn to the list of changes that Meredith has recited. Further exploration showed that not only had Meredith moved to another state away from Don but she had also lost her sex drive and was finding men repulsive. She was in a deep depression and simply wanted to be left alone. It was evident that the state of affairs between Meredith and Don was not simply that he was getting close to someone else; Meredith was actively pushing him away. Clearly there was much self-exploration that Meredith needed to engage in before she could take any action.

In the early sessions of the group, it is important to help group members focus on their own internal reactions so that they become aware of how the cancer affects them, along with any implications this may have for the members individually or for the group process. As your group members become more aware of their internal response to having cancer and the implications it has for their lives and for those they care about, they can begin to examine their coping strategies. Thus, as the treatment progresses, the strategy should move increasingly toward the facilitation of active coping strategies. While it is always appropriate to encourage the expression and exploration of thoughts and feelings, there should be a gradual movement toward the facilitation of active, problem-focused coping.

Problems that arise as a result of cancer often seem huge and overwhelming and, as a result, patients can feel that there is little they can do to deal with the problem. This feeling arises because of the tendency to think that one must solve the problem in its entirety. Also, some of the problems may seem unresolvable, such as the fear of dying a painful death or becoming completely dependent on others for one's physical care. To deal with these large and difficult problems, we help our patients to break the problem down into smaller, more manageable pieces. Once the problem is broken down, we ask them to focus on one of these pieces and to see if there is anything they can do about that one piece. Often to their surprise, they find that there is.

STIMULATE INTERACTION

The best group sessions are the most interactive ones, in which all members participate even though the discussion might overtly be about one or two of them. In the example above, it may be evident that these particular group members had no difficulty interacting with each other. It was the quality of their interactions, however, that was a concern. Many of the women in this group had strong personalities. The group culture that had developed and that the therapists now had to work to undo was one where members interrupted each other in order to make their point, often not responding to the comments of others and occasionally breaking out into several conversations at once. The task of the therapists was to facilitate an interactional style that included actively listening to one another and taking the time to reflect on their own reactions before blurting them out and charging forth in some other direction. In other groups there may be an opposite problem where members need to be drawn out so that they can be active participants.

For many patients, being in a group where they talk about feelings is a novel experience and can be uncomfortable at first. Such members may need extra support and assistance. For example, a good strategy with silent members is to turn to them occasionally and ask: "Have any thoughts or feelings come up for you as you've been listening to the discussion?" or, "What do you think about what has been said?" or, "Do any of these issues pertain to your life?" In terms of group interaction, the aim is to develop a culture where all members participate, actively listen, and respond to one another in a supportive manner.

KEEP THE FOCUS ON CANCER

Finally, another aspect of the culture you should seek to establish early on in your group is that the focus of the group is cancer. This may seem self-evident, but you will be surprised to find that after the first couple of sessions, your members may feel that they have exhausted the subject of cancer and are ready to move on to other topics. This occurs with individuals who are not used to exploring their internal experiences, and as a result, once they have told their stories, they feel that there is not much more to be said.

At the same time, it is important to remember that cancer affects one's entire life, including relationships, work, and play. Consequently, it will be necessary to deal with topics that are not explicitly about cancer. As you do so, however, you should make a point of linking the issue to cancer. For example, if long-standing relationship problems are being discussed, you can make the following types of intervention: "Has having cancer exacerbated these problems in any way?" or "This must make you feel awfully alone with your cancer."

During the early sessions of your group, the central goal is to establish a culture that is conducive to working on the challenge of learning to live with cancer. During this stage of the group, you will need to play an active role in establishing the appropriate culture. Once it is established, you will find that you will need to pay less attention to these factors because to that extent the group will be self-led. For instance, there will be less of a need to facilitate the expression of support among group members; they will do this naturally. Instead, you can shift your focus to the work of deepening the exploration of issues that arise for your members as they live with this disease.

CONCLUSION

In this chapter we have provided an overview of the issues involved in forming a supportive-expressive cancer group as well as during the group's early sessions. Attending to how you recruit patients, ensuring that both you and the patient have similar goals and that the patient is a good fit for the group, is the first important step. Once you have carefully selected your patients and prepared them for the group, then you will be well placed to set the group on the proper track. While there is much to consider in this beginning phase of your group, paying close and careful attention to these details is your greatest guarantee for a successful group experience for everyone.

CHAPTER 4

Treatment Strategies and Options for the Therapist

Typically, supportive-expressive cancer groups are composed of psychologically healthy individuals who happen to be dealing with a major life crisis. Their reason for involvement in the group is not to resolve long-standing intrapsychic issues but to deal with their illness. You will find that many, if not most, of the people in your group are individuals who prior to their cancer were functioning well at home and at work. As a result of the cancer, however, they are faced with a stressor that would be a crisis for anyone. Consequently, the group's purpose is not personality change, but rather to help patients adjust to their new circumstances and cope with the concomitant psychological, social, and physical changes they are experiencing.

Contrary to practice in traditional psychotherapy groups, we encourage outside contact between group members. We believe that the group is not simply a social microcosm for the patient, but serves as a buffer against the traumatic effects of facing cancer alone. Thus, the more group members can support each other inside and outside the group, the greater the buffering effect.

THE BASIC TREATMENT STRATEGIES

There are six basic strategies we use throughout the life of the group to facilitate members in dealing with their disease and its psychological, social, and physical consequences:

1. maintain the focus on cancer,
2. help group members explore their personal experience in having cancer,
3. work in the here-and-now,
4. encourage active coping,
5. promote supportive interactions among group members, and
6. use relaxation and guided imagery to deal with pain and to work on issues that arise because of the cancer.

MAINTAIN THE
FOCUS ON CANCER

It may seem obvious and even unnecessary to say that the focus of these groups should remain on cancer; after all, isn't that why these groups were formed? While it is true that the point of these groups is to talk about cancer, the fact that special groups have to be formed for this purpose indicates that talking about cancer is not an easy matter.

Speaking about cancer and the myriad ways it affects an individual's life and sense of the future can be threatening. As a result, there is often a tendency to get sidetracked onto other less threatening topics. When this happens, it is the responsibility of the leader to redirect the discussion back to cancer. Typically, whatever the "noncancer" subject matter may be, it is somehow related to cancer. In fact, the noncancer topic is often *on* topic, although this may be covert and thus not apparent to the members. It is up to the group leader to point out the link to cancer so that the group members can speak more explicitly and directly about the particular cancer issue. At other times, the noncancer topic may be a way of avoiding some important cancer-related issue. This too should be brought out into the open so that the members can be helped to deal with the troubling matter.

Explore Digressions. During one of our metastatic breast cancer groups the discussion turned to the topic of children and how open and self-disclosing cancer patients should be about the disease. This talk led one member, Marleen, to discuss problems that her brother was having with his daughters. Marleen went on at length about their difficulties with each other and the extent to which it bothered her. It was clear that Marleen was preoccupied with her brother's problems, but it was not so clear what this had to do with Marleen's own struggle with cancer.

Even though Marleen was not talking about an issue related to cancer, the group members and leaders felt the importance of this issue for her and yet were at a loss about how to help her or how to redirect the discussion to cancer-related issues.

This type of situation is not uncommon and can be particularly challenging for the novice leader.

The way in which this particular situation got resolved was that one of the leaders asked the question, "Marleen, why is this so potent for you?" Although Marleen was unable to answer this question in a way that made the link to her own cancer experience, the question began to percolate within the minds of others in the group.

Eventually, the members began to offer possible answers for Marleen. They talked about their own struggles with unfinished business and the desire to resolve these issues before dying. For some, there were times when resolution was beyond their control and the challenge came in learning how to let go. This discussion enabled Marleen to reflect upon her overinvolvement in her brother's problem and to realize that this was a problem only he could solve.

Redirect Discussion.   Another possible intervention would have been the following: "Marleen, I noticed that a few minutes ago we were talking about how much to tell children about one's illness and I am wondering if this is a concern of yours with your own children." The strategy with this intervention is to simply ignore the diversion and to refocus the discussion back to the original topic. This type of intervention is useful when it appears that the shift away from cancer is simply to divert the discussion and not necessarily because there is a more important issue to discuss. Diversions often occur because the topic at hand is too threatening. We have found that it is more productive to simply redirect the discussion back to the threatening topic than it is to point out the defensive shift away from the topic.

Explore Emotion.   Another approach is to inquire about the group members' emotional response to the subject that had been diverted—for example, "I noticed that we have moved away from the discussion about talking to children about illness and I'm wondering if that discussion brings up difficult feelings for anyone." As we will discuss later in this chapter and in Chapter 6, focusing on group members' emotional responses is an effective way of getting to the heart of the issues.

Observe Process.   Sometimes you may find that the group does not seem to be able to keep the focus on cancer. It is important to help the group discover what they might be avoiding. For instance, this can happen after an especially difficult meeting and may be a way of avoiding important but difficult material. In such a case it can be useful to say something like "Last week we talked about some hard issues and I'm wondering if any you have anything more you want to say about it." Or, "Last week was a hard session and I'm wondering if any of you have thought any more about it during the week or had any reactions to it."

Sometimes there may be some important issue that the group as a whole is trying to avoid, such as having learned that one of the group members has just received some bad news about her condition. In such a case you might say, "I can't help but notice that we are talking about things that are not at all cancer-related. It makes me wonder if we're doing that because we are afraid to talk about what is really on our mind, which is how we feel about Mary's bad news."

Empathize.   There are times when you might not discern any particular reason for why the discussion is not cancer-related and it is simply a matter of your somehow shifting the discussion to cancer. Doing this can often feel challenging in that there might not be any obvious way to do this. The best way to approach these kinds of situations is to silently ask yourself, "How might this be related to cancer or impact someone who has cancer?" Listening through this filter usually stimulates ideas that you can then use to shift the discussion. For instance, "You know, Megan, while you've been talking about your difficulties with your husband, I've found myself thinking how difficult it must be to have cancer and to feel that your husband is too busy to listen to you." Or, "What is it like to have this problem to cope with at the same time that you are also coping with cancer?" When all else fails, you can simply ask "Does anyone have any cancer-related concerns they would like to talk about tonight?"

HELP GROUP MEMBERS EXPLORE
THEIR CANCER EXPERIENCE

A diagnosis of cancer evokes a multitude of difficult issues and feelings, many of which are often actively avoided. The avoidance or denial of threatening thoughts and feelings can provide a measure of relief in the short term. However, in the long term it has deleterious consequences. First and foremost, it reinforces the profound sense of isolation and aloneness that patients feel when diagnosed with cancer. Furthermore, it intensifies the belief that these difficult issues and feelings are unmanageable. The end result is often feelings of despair, helplessness, and a sense of futility.

There are a variety of reasons that a patient may want to suppress and control troublesome thoughts and feelings. One reason stems from the popular belief that a consistently positive attitude is necessary to promote healing. Many cancer patients have come to fear negative or painful feelings and refuse to acknowledge negative thoughts. The concern is that having these thoughts or feelings will cause the cancer to recur, spread, or in some way interfere with healing. There are two problems with this viewpoint. One is that in the cancer patient's desperation to promote healing, there is a tendency to repress negative feelings, which unfortunately does not make them go away, but in fact is likely to make them worse. The second problem is that if there is a recurrence or some kind of disease progression, the cancer patient feels blamed and held responsible, a clearly counterproductive outcome. This latter attitude has regrettably become rampant in our society. One of our patients reported being asked by a friend who, upon hearing about her recurrence, asked why she had wanted her cancer to spread.

Another common fear that leads to cancer patients' attempts to control thoughts and feelings is a fear of being overwhelmed, or of overwhelming others. The group provides an ideal environment for testing these beliefs. One of the more important lessons for cancer patients is to learn that they can tolerate their own emotions. The role of the therapist is critical here. The leaders must convey a sense that the leaders themselves can tolerate any thoughts or feelings that arise in the group. This is a prerequisite to group members taking the risk of exploring their own frightening feelings and thoughts.

Following a memorial service for one of the group members, the group had a painful discussion about the death of this member as well as other deaths that had occurred in their group. At one point, the group leader turned to Megan and inquired about her statement that she had been thinking of Jane, a member who had died several months previously, and what thoughts she had. Megan snapped at the leader, saying, "None of your business!"

Believing that Megan's outburst covered up some difficult feelings she had, he asked, "Can you tell me what you are angry about?" Because he faced her anger directly and inquired in an open and nondefensive manner, Megan could see that the group leader would not be overwhelmed by his own feelings or by hers. This gave Megan the courage to believe that her thoughts and feelings were tolerable to both herself and to others. Megan admitted that she snapped at him and didn't want to talk because she was reluctant to let herself feel how sad she was. Having said this enabled her to express her deep pain over the loss of these vital women.

This example demonstrates that by facing the issue directly and openly, the leader permits the group members to do the same.

Facilitate Expression and Exploration of Feelings.   Expressing and exploring difficult thoughts and feelings require the patient to enter into a disturbing and sometimes terrifying realm of experience. What if he or she were to become engulfed by that experience? It is such fantasizing that frightens patients. Consequently, as important as being able to enter into the experience is being able to detach from it in order to reflect upon it.

Isabel was a woman with advanced breast cancer who was phobic about dying. She described how she would awaken in the middle of the night gripped with terror at the realization that she was going to die. Her phobia predated the cancer and ironically she found that since having cancer it had diminished somewhat for her. During one meeting her phobia was the topic of discussion and the group leader asked her if she would like to work on it. Isabel expressed her fear at doing this. "What do you think would happen if you looked a little more closely at the thought of dying?" the therapist asked. "I don't know. . . . I guess . . . I guess, maybe I'm afraid that I would die just by looking at it." "Do you think that is really possible?" the therapist asked. "Well, probably not," she replied. "How about if we just look at one small part of what you fear about dying?" she was asked. Isabel agreed and the therapist proceeded to help her imagine that she was dying. She was instructed to identify the first thing that came to her mind and then to stop there so that they could talk about it. Isabel did as instructed and discovered that she was afraid of being alone during the dying process.

This exercise enabled Isabel to enter briefly into the feared experience and then to step back so that she could look at the thoughts and feelings that emerged. Several things were accomplished. One is that it taught her that she would not be overwhelmed by the experience. It also taught her that she could control the experience. Finally, it enabled her to extract a piece of what concerned her and to think about what she could do about it. In fact, the entire group benefited from this process. During the remainder of the session the group discussed what they can do to ensure that during the process of dying they are cared for in the manner that they desire.

The crucial aspects of the intervention were that the therapist:

- Identified the issue
- Absorbed and stayed with the emotion
- Explored it further
- Helped the patient understand problems that were sources of the emotion
- Pursued her finding ways of coping more actively with the problem
- Maintained an empathic stance with the patient throughout
- Involved the whole group in the process

As we have seen, the therapist plays an important role in helping the patient modulate the extent to which he or she enters into the feared experience. The group leader's warmth and empathic support are also crucial for helping the patient to tolerate the feelings. The leader can function as a lifeline by helping the patient to detach from these feelings if they become intolerable. Fortunately, however, there is a natural and adaptive tendency to allow oneself to experience only as much as can be tolerated, and in dealing with any extremely painful material, it can only be done in small doses. Thus, for most people, both the patient and the facilitator can count on this built-in defense mechanism to protect the patient from being engulfed by terrifying thoughts and feelings. The patient will naturally pull back if it becomes too threatening.

Stepping back from the experience is important if the patient is to learn from it. The goal is to help the patient develop a more adaptive perspective on this aspect of self and her ability to cope. Often other group members will spontaneously become involved in this stage of the exploration. They will offer words of understanding and encouragement or draw on their own experiences to illustrate coping strategies that have worked for them. If this does not occur spontaneously, the group leaders can explicitly elicit feedback from the group.

Maintain Specific and Concrete Focus.   It is not uncommon for patients to speak about cancer in abstract and impersonal ways. This is a way of speaking about what is troubling them and yet it also gives the illusion of keeping cancer at a distance.

Thus, helping members focus on personal and specific issues is an important principle in supportive-expressive group therapy.

There is a natural tendency when talking about difficulties in life to speak in general and abstract terms: "I'm feeling so depressed about my life. Cancer seems to be consuming everything." This statement is difficult to work with. It is global and sweeping, providing little indication of the ways in which the cancer interferes in the patient's life. A place to begin with such a statement is to ask what kinds of situations the person has in mind when he or she says the cancer is all-consuming. The leader should help the member to be more specific and, whenever possible, to find out if it is being experienced in some way right now in the group. The more concrete, personal, and rooted in the present the person can be when working on a problem, the more the patient can access the underlying feelings, beliefs, and assumptions that have contributed to the problem. Working on a specific problem that is being experienced in the moment also provides the group member or members the opportunity to resolve the problem by enacting the solution in the present.

> *Elizabeth's metastatic breast cancer was slowly progressing. She had been away for several weeks and when she returned she reported that there had been a spread of her cancer and that she faced the prospect of indefinite chemotherapy. On top of that she was feeling unsupported by people. This vague reference to "people" led the group leader to ask if she could be more specific. Elizabeth responded by talking about her husband, who was in the middle of a major project, thereby making him more unavailable. After some exploration of this issue, the leader decided to shift the focus away from her relationship with the husband and toward the group. She asked, "Do you feel that you are getting the support you want from us?"*
>
> *Somewhat hesitantly, Elizabeth replied that she was feeling concerned that the group would not support her desire to refuse chemotherapy and that ultimately she feared they would abandon her. After hearing the feedback and unconditional support of the group members, the group leaders helped her to recognize how her long-standing fear of abandonment had resulted in her keeping her thoughts and feelings to herself, thereby depriving her of the opportunity to get the support she craved.*

Helping Elizabeth become more specific about feeling unsupported and relating this issue directly to her experience in the group helped Elizabeth to see not only what beliefs were underlying these feelings but also what she was doing to contribute to her not getting the support she needed.

Encourage Group Involvement. When we are facilitating the exploration of patients' cancer experiences, it is also important to encourage the involvement of all group members. Certainly, there will be an ebb and flow between focusing on a single individual's issues and inviting all group members to examine an issue as it pertains to each of them. Group therapy should not be a series of individual therapies with a group of witnesses. Instead, there should be a continual interplay between focusing on a particular individual's issues and relating these to everyone else in the group. Thus, one of the skills that you must learn is how to take an individual's unique issues and apply it to the group as a whole. This involves listening for themes.

> *Sophia was a stylish woman who took great pleasure in dressing well and looking good. She also had metastatic breast cancer and as a result of chemotherapy had developed lymphedema in one of her arms. She had done everything she could to reduce the swelling in her arm but to no avail. Because of her concern with her appearance and her frustration that the swelling in her arm was not going down, she came to group one day quite distraught. She spoke at length about what she has been doing to reduce the swelling and how having this swollen arm has affected what she can wear and how she feels about herself. The group leader then made the following intervention: "As I listen to what you are saying about how unhappy you are with having lymphedema and its effect on your appearance, I wonder if you are also saying something else. Having cancer has meant that you have had to give up parts of your identity, of how you see yourself. I'm wondering if we can talk about what it has been like for you and for others in the group to give up parts of yourself because of cancer."*

This intervention generalized the issue so that all group members could relate to the discussion and examine their own unique experience on the effect of cancer on their identity.

Thus, in helping group members explore their cancer experience, you should also encourage them to speak both personally and specifically. Pay attention to emotions that emerge; they can inform you about the direction in which the exploration should be facilitated. If the emotions and thoughts seem overwhelming to the patients, help them break the issue down into manageable pieces. Finding that there is a piece of the problem that they can handle also serves the function of giving them hope regarding their ability to cope with whatever comes their way. Finally, listen for broader themes that can be applied to the group as a whole so that everyone can deepen their understanding of their own experience.

WORKING IN THE HERE-AND-NOW

Working in the here-and-now is one of the active ingredients in group therapy. It is also a way of interacting that is foreign to most people and thus is something that patients need to be taught to do and to value. Thus, from the outset it is important for you to pay attention to the here-and-now so that you can begin to comment on it and to work with it and thereby communicate its central place in the group work.

As with any form of therapy, accessing and working with immediate experience is far more potent than dealing with abstractions or experiences in the past. It is inevitable, of course, that members will bring in material from the outside. They will talk about experiences from their distant or recent past, and in fact, it is important that they bring in this kind of material. For cancer patients, talking about the history of their disease, its diagnosis and treatment, and the broader context of their lives is not only unavoidable but essential. The job of the therapist is to shift the focus of these discussions to the here-and-now. This is always possible because any experiences that are brought in from the past elicit emotions in the present. At the same time, they may also have implications for how one chooses to be in the future, as demonstrated in the following example.

> Venita, a very ill breast cancer patient, came to group one day not looking well at all. She attributed this in a rather pressured and long discussion to inflammation she was experiencing as a result of radiation to her hip. As the therapist listened, he was aware that although she was describing her present condition, she was doing so in a detached manner. Further he felt that she was indirectly asking for support. As a way to shift the focus to the here-and-now and to help her speak more directly about what she wants, he asked, "Venita, is there anything we can do to help you right now?" Venita began to cry and to talk about how hurt she had been that she had been in bed for a week and no one from the group had called her. This led to a fruitful discussion among the group members about the distancing messages they feel they get from Venita and how this had made many of them reluctant to reach out to her.

This discussion about the here-and-now issues between the group members and Venita had many benefits for both her and the rest of the group. An important outcome for Venita was that it helped her to recognize how she needed to change her behavior so that she more clearly stated her needs and desires to those around her.

Activation.   Yalom (1995) stresses that working in the here-and-now has two components, one of which is *activation* of the here-and-now. Activation of the here-and-now occurs naturally. We cannot deny that at any given moment each of us has an immediate experience; for instance, right now you are embedded in a particular experience as you are reading this book. The role of the therapist is to help the group members attend to their immediate experience. This has the potential to be quite powerful. For example, asking the group members, "How do you feel listening to Amy's story?" provides an opportunity for the members to turn their focus inward.

It is not unusual for patients to discover something about themselves when they are asked for their reactions to hearing someone's story. It also frequently results in an outpouring of support for the member who has just shared his or her experience. Facilitating the expression of patients' here-and-now experience enables patients to discover that their own internal response is both acceptable and important. It greatly diminishes the sense of being alone with the disease. Thus, focusing on the here-and-now presents opportunities for each person to express his or her thoughts and feelings and to provide support for each other.

Although there is always a here-and-now experience, there are times when you may want to deliberately activate the here-and-now. This strategy is one that you should employ only when you think it would be particularly appropriate and useful. For example, we have patients who are so self-reliant and independent that they find it extremely difficult, if not impossible, to ask for help in any form. However, having cancer places them in the uncomfortable position of needing assistance from time to time. Asking such a patient to identify some way in which the group or particular members could help her, followed by an instruction to make that request of the group right now, will result in a powerful activation of the patient's internal conflict. Helping the patient work through that internal response in the context of a supportive group environment can be particularly helpful. She may find that she worries about how others will view her if she is dependent.

This concern can be addressed directly by asking the group what they think of her as a result of her asking for help. She may be aware that she finds it difficult to believe anyone will follow through on her request for support. Or she may discover that she feels like a failure because she needs help and can't do it on her own. All of these are issues that can be effectively addressed in a group context.

Illumination of Process.   The second component Yalom speaks of involves the illumination of process. This involves helping the group members to reflect on and to understand their interactions in the group. This type of intervention is particularly useful for group psychotherapy where the purpose of the group is to facilitate personality change. In supportive-expressive cancer groups, however, the goal is not personality change but rather to help patients feel less alone with their illness, to improve social and family support, to integrate a changed self- and body image, to improve coping skills, and to help patients achieve greater emotional expression. Thus, for supportive-expressive groups, process statements are made in the service of facilitating the goals unique to this form of treatment.

Often members are not aware of their own internal experience, even though it may be coloring both their perceptions and their experience. Asking such simple questions as, "What is coming up for you as you listen to Mary talk?" or "I'm wondering what you are feeling right now as you're telling us about having to wait for the results of the MRI" are often all that is required to shift the focus to the experiential. Sometimes you may find it necessary to give your perception of what the patient might be experiencing internally. This is especially true for patients who are not accustomed to attending to their emotions. For example, "You seem so sad as you are speaking." Even if you are wrong, for most people such a statement will force them to direct their focus inward in order to determine whether it is sadness that is being felt or something else.

Group leaders should always attend to the underlying group process. Often patients find indirect and sometimes unconscious ways of expressing their feelings, needs, or concerns. This is particularly true if the thought or feeling is threatening. In such circumstances the group leaders may need to take an active role in helping the patient identify and express his or her true feelings.

In the fourth meeting of a primary breast cancer group, one of the members, Wendy, speaks repeatedly about the anxiety she has been feeling because of the cancer. Lori, an-

other group member, becomes engaged in helping Wendy find a way to manage her anx-
iety. For some reason, however, the group leaders remain relatively uninvolved in the
discussion. As the discussion between Wendy and Lori continues, Wendy eventually
says to Lori, "You're good, Lori. Maybe I'll go see you in therapy."

This statement is an indirect message to the group leaders who have not been providing the support that Wendy seeks. At this point it is important for the group leaders to help Wendy voice her true feelings about the apparent lack of support from the leaders. Once this is acknowledged, Wendy may be able to talk about what she needs from the leaders as well as other authority figures in her life. Working this through with Wendy may require therapist transparency. Was there something in how Wendy was speaking about her anxiety that kept the leaders from responding? What kinds of feelings were activated in the leaders that prevented their response? A genuine response to Wendy about how she is experienced by the group leaders may help Wendy see the ways in which she prevents people from supporting her. Illuminating the process in this manner not only provides insight into the patient's experience but also communicates that no subject is too frightening to broach.

Yalom suggests that one type of process illumination be used judiciously—process interventions that focus solely on the "mass group phenomenon," where the focus of the intervention is on the group as a whole. Yalom recommends using this type of intervention only in circumstances when there seems to be an obstacle that is interfering with the group work. For example, we have a group that is co-led by two experienced group leaders, although one of these leaders is perceived by the members to be the primary leader. From time to time, the primary leader is unable to attend. What we have noticed is that often when this leader is absent, the group engages in more superficial chatter or focuses on technical medical treatment issues and does not speak at a more personal and meaningful level.

In such a situation, an intervention like the following may facilitate the group to speak about the issues that are really concerning them: "I've noticed that today has been an unusual meeting for us as we've been spending most of our time talking about treatment issues. I'm wondering if we could step back from the discussion for a minute and talk about today's meeting. Do you feel like you are getting what you need today? Are there other concerns that you would rather be talking about?" Depending on where this takes the group, the intervention might be followed up with a more direct question regarding the "primary" leader's absence: "Do you think Dr. Smith's absence has had an influence on the tone of today's discussion?" This question may provide an opportunity for the group to address the topic that they have been working hard to avoid—their concern that the "secondary" leader cannot provide them with what they need.

To facilitate an experiential exploration requires helping members to track their internal emotional experience as it unfolds. This can be a challenging endeavor, particularly if the topic is one that is being defended against.

In one of our metastatic breast cancer groups, a forty-year-old woman, Ellen, announced at the beginning of a group that she had finally made an appointment to have "that nasty cough checked." She exuded a nervous, hyper energy. After completing this announcement, Ellen said, "So that's all I wanted to say. We can let someone else talk now." Viewing this comment and her manner as a red flag, the leaders encouraged her to talk about how she was feeling about having the test. "Oh, I'm okay. It will just be good to have it over. But really, I'm okay." To which the leader responded, "You sounded a little choked when you said you'll be glad to have it over. Can you tell us what comes up for you when you say that?" "Oh, I'm just nervous, that's all," Ellen replied. "What kinds of thoughts or images are passing through your mind?" the leader asked.

This active probing and concerted effort to help Ellen attend to her internal experience as it was unfolding enabled her to speak about the terror that was gripping her and had been consuming her over the last few days. Ellen's fear was that the cancer had metastasized, that this would require going on chemotherapy, and that it was the beginning of the end for her. Being immersed in these feelings, she was able finally to cry. Following the release of these pent-up emotions, she was also able to step back from the experience and learn from it. She realized that over the past several days she had been caught up in frenetic activity as a way to avoid dealing with her fears. What Ellen discovered during the next week was that she found herself to be in a much better position to cope with her situation. Often, real discoveries about personal experience will only occur if the patient is in touch with and explores the experience as it unfolds.

Similarly, working in the context of a member's relationship with other members in the group provides an opportunity to deal experientially and interactively with problems. A common problem for people afflicted with cancer is that they feel alone and cast out. Cancer is an isolating experience in that it immediately sets the individual apart and it can seem that there are few who fully understand. In a supportive-expressive group the cancer patient is presented with an opportunity to work through these feelings of isolation via his or her relationships with other group members.

> *In one metastatic breast cancer group, a patient, Beth, said that she had something "small" that she had wanted to bring up the previous week but didn't because she felt that there were other more important concerns in the group. She described having received the results of a medical report and noting that one of the laboratory tests indicated a rise in a measure of her liver function. After reading the report, she called her physician to inquire about it. His response was that this change was not something she needs to worry about. Beth continued to feel worried, however, and approached two other physicians, as well as other individuals in her life who had some knowledge of this test. In spite of everyone's assurances, she continued to worry. In particular, she said, she wanted to get this cleared up before she went home to visit her family and friends, whom she had not seen for three years.*
>
> *In response to Beth's anxiety, various women in the group gave whatever bit of knowledge they had about this test, until finally another member said, "Beth, you're really worried about going home and having everyone see you like this, aren't you?" To which Beth started to cry. "I want them to see me as Beth, not Beth-with-cancer." This she realized was the key issue, not the medical tests. Furthermore, it was not a trivial concern as several members were quick to point out to her. Consequently, she also realized that she tends to minimize her concerns in comparison to the worries of others.*

The job of the leader is to help the group move beyond the abstract, intellectual level toward the experiential. This can only be accomplished by working in the here-and-now. It is useful to keep in mind that whatever the issue under discussion, your group members are always having some kind of internal reaction. By shifting the discussion to this here-and-now experience, you can help your group members access their emotional response to the topic. Working in the here-and-now is a potent strategy for helping patients get to the heart of the matter.

PROMOTE SUPPORTIVE INTERACTIONS AMONG GROUP MEMBERS

A fundamental goal of any group therapy is to bring a group of people together with the intention that they interact and ultimately form significant relationships. In supportive-expressive groups we take this goal a step further by aiming for the development of supportive relationships. This is almost immediately accomplished by being in the presence of others who share similar experiences. In virtually every cancer group we have led, patients have commented on the support that is felt from being in a group with other cancer patients. It is clear that our group members derive enormous benefit by spending time with each other. The common refrain is that the group is unlike any other place they have—here they do not need to explain what they mean when they talk about their cancer, its treatment, or what it feels like to live with this disease.

Even though the simple fact of being in a cancer support group is helpful, there is a definite role for the group leaders to play in facilitating supportive interaction among group members. We view group support as involving interaction among members where there is the opportunity for open expression, for giving as well as receiving support, and ultimately for diminishing feelings of isolation. The therapist's role is to facilitate the development of a supportive, accepting, and open atmosphere where patients can share all aspects of their experience. It is particularly important in early meetings that the leaders set the tone by offering warmth and understanding. Supportive behaviors and attitudes can be continually encouraged by the therapist's modeling of empathy and support.

Although it is important for the therapist to be supportive, it is even more important to facilitate members supporting each other. In this respect the therapist can take an active role. For instance, if someone has revealed something painful, the therapist might ask the group what it was like to hear this. This kind of question frequently leads to supportive statements on the part of other members or, alternatively, it can lead to others revealing similar pains. Whatever the outcome, both of these responses are likely to make the patient feel supported and less alone with his or her pain.

Mobilizing the Group to Provide Support.   Mutual support comes from sharing meaningful personal experiences with others, as well as common concerns. It entails both receiving support and offering support to other group members. This fosters the development of rapport and mutual caring, which generally extends beyond the parameters of group meetings. The potential for providing support outside the group increases as the members begin to share information and common experiences and to help each other with both practical and emotional support.

Providing support, however, is not always as simple as it seems. In the following example the group leader drew on the group members to help one member, Frances, resolve her concerns about whether she had been supportive enough to another member.

Frances talked about how worried she was about Liz, who was both absent from group and quite ill. Frances described talking to Liz on the phone and asking her if there was anything she could do to be helpful. Liz thanked her but said no. When talking to the group about the conversation, Frances seemed bothered and uncertain about what she had done, which was to accept Liz's response at face value. She expressed regret that she didn't simply show up at Liz's door in order to be with her. To help Frances resolve these mixed feelings, the group leader asked the members how they would have felt if Frances had responded to them as she did to Liz. One woman remarked that she would have felt wonderful that Frances had shown she cared by asking if she could be of help and that she also respected her boundaries by listening to her when she said no. Another woman had a very different reaction, which was that she would have felt frightened by Frances's concern. Hearing these two very different responses enabled Frances to appreciate the enormous individuality in people's reactions, including her own. This allowed her to give herself permission to listen to her own internal voice as a way of discerning what is right for her and for how she wants to relate to others.

Another example that illustrates the complexity of support occurred in a brief primary breast cancer group.

The group leader turned to one of the older members, Rita, and commented that she had not spoken all night. Rita replied that similar to what others had been saying, she has had her scares and that she tries to deal with them on a day-to-day basis. However, she feels that she has not had the hard knocks that others have had and so has had an ordinary life. The group leader then asked if being in the group brought up other feelings.

This was a good question because it had the potential to shift the focus to more difficult issues, which is precisely what happened.

Rita talked about how she wonders about who one should turn to when these "scares" happen. She then described her surgeon telling her she had cancer and promptly dismissing her from his office. Having described this incident she shifted to talking about how doctors should treat their patients by, for instance, referring them to support groups.

Rita's story was a poignant one and needed to be pursued. This was immediately apparent because Rita began to cry. Because of their discomfort and out of a desire to be supportive, other group members reacted by talking about their experiences with their surgeons and how bad they felt for Rita. While this type of support can be very helpful, it was premature at this point. The focus of the group should have been on helping Rita to sit with her feelings and to explore them. The group leaders are crucial at this point. They should ignore what other members are saying and return to Rita, asking her to talk about what happened and how she feels.

> *Eventually the focus returned to Rita, but she still did not get the help she needed. The members encouraged her to change her doctor and to tell them his name. Then the focus shifted again to people talking about their various experiences with their doctors. There was a discussion about getting second opinions and the flak some of them got for doing that. Unfortunately, the end result for Rita was that she had feelings stirred up but was not helped to deal with them. Thus, she ended the session crying throughout the concluding hypnosis exercise.*

This example illustrates the important role that the group leaders have in ensuring that members get the kind of support they need. There are times when it can be very helpful to have group members share their own experience as a means of providing support. There are other times when what feels most supportive is to have people listen and to let the person know that they care.

Sharing the experience of having cancer and of being in the group involves expression of one's internal experience and is necessarily interactive. All communication within a group affects other group members, whether or not the members acknowledge it. The therapist's task is to facilitate the expression of these effects and to encourage direct communication between members.

> *One group member, Pam, spoke about the difficulty she experiences, now that she is sick, in dealing with her elderly mother. It seemed that her mother could not accommodate to the idea that her daughter was also in a position of needing support. Lillian, an elderly member of the group, suddenly broke in complaining about her son's busy schedule. Following up on this apparent non sequitur, the leader asked Lillian if she had any reactions to Pam's story about her mother. This enabled Lillian to speak about her feelings of guilt that her son has to take so much time away from his work to help her now that she has become ill. This led to a fruitful interaction between Lillian and Pam about their respective roles as mother and daughter and how it has been affected by breast cancer.*

The facilitation of supportive interaction among group members is an ongoing and essential role that the therapist plays. Communication should proceed in all possible directions and not solely through the group leaders. The direct expression of members' thoughts and feelings to each other is critical for the establishment of trust and mutual support.

ENCOURAGE ACTIVE COPING

When patients are diagnosed with a chronic and potentially life-threatening disease such as cancer, it is not uncommon for them to feel overwhelmed, helpless, and hopeless. They may feel that there is very little they can do to improve their situation, so they give up in resignation, taking a passive or avoidant orientation toward their illness. If they are feeling overwhelmed by the enormity of the problem they face, they may simply avoid dealing with it or may even deny what is happening. We have heard many stories of patients who upon hearing the diagnosis suddenly "leave their bodies" and feel as though it was happening to someone else. Or they might simply stop hearing what is being told to them. (This is one reason it is useful to either have a family member or friend with the patient when this kind of information is being delivered or to tape-record the conversation so that they can eventually hear the information.) We have also heard of patients who were informed that they had cancer and then went on for months as though nothing had changed, only to have the information finally register. Clearly these are not adaptive coping strategies.

The types of coping that have been found to be most helpful are active problem-focused coping strategies (Fawzy, Cousins et al., 1990). Thus, in our groups we try to facilitate coping strategies that involve taking positive steps toward improving their quality of life, understanding their illness and its effect upon them, and taking appropriate steps to deal directly with their disease. Patients are encouraged to get more involved in their treatment and in monitoring their disease. This includes such actions as learning about the illness, paying close attention to symptoms, getting regular breast or prostate exams, working collaboratively with their doctor, or seeking second opinions if need be. For emotional or interpersonal issues, they are encouraged to seek the support they want from people around them, both inside and outside the group. While active coping strategies are encouraged in our groups, we are also mindful of the proper timing when we shift toward a discussion of strategies patients can use to cope with their illness.

Avoiding Premature Resolution.   Although active coping is clearly a goal we
have for our patients, it is important that the leader not shift the focus to active coping prematurely. This issue, discussed briefly in Chapter 3, is a problem that we often see in novice group leaders. We suspect that it comes out of
the anxiety that gets simulated in novice group leaders who often mistakenly
feel that it is their responsibility to solve the patient's problem. Not knowing
what else to do and unconsciously seeking to quell their own anxiety, novice
leaders will often turn to the only strategy they can think of. This is usually
to help the patient think about what they can do to make the problem go
away. While we agree that it is certainly the group leaders' responsibility to
help the patient solve the problem, in our experience shifting prematurely to
discuss coping strategies is usually not very helpful.

It is also important to note that the pressure that the group leaders feel to
solve the problem is a pressure that other group members are likely to feel
when someone in their group is distressed about a problem. It is human nature to want to jump in and fix things. Thus, the group leaders should be
aware of both their own internal need to solve the problem as well as monitoring the tendency of the group to offer advice as a way to help a patient
with a problem. This is necessary so that premature discussions of coping
strategies do not derail members from getting to the heart of the problem.

Let's return again to the example of Meredith.

*Meredith is the breast cancer patient who introduced her partner of five years to a fe-
male friend and expressed anger about his wanting to talk to Meredith about his feelings
for the friend. She was also angry and depressed about being "the cancer person." The
focus shifted once more to Meredith when another member, Janet, decided to be unusually self-revealing in order to illustrate how Meredith should try to find pleasure in her
life. Janet described going into an arts-and-crafts shop one day and feeling an overwhelming sense of well-being. She went on to say that she gets great pleasure out of arts
and crafts and makes a point of taking the time to do her craft. This was Janet's way of
offering advice to Meredith about what she should do to make herself feel better. Meredith responded, "My depression is coming from the fact that I don't want to do anything.
Everything that used to give me meaning doesn't any longer." At this point another
member commented that Meredith sounded hopeless. Meredith responded, "I am beyond feeling hopeless. I don't care enough to feel hopeless."*

*(As a footnote, when patients sound this depressed, it is essential that you assess
for suicide risk and, if necessary, refer for more intensive psychotherapy and pharma-
cotherapy.)*

Meredith continued to get a lot of support and suggestions from the group. The level of advice giving that occurs is often directly proportional to the amount of distress that is expressed, as was true in this case. It further illustrates that when anxiety gets stimulated in the listener, it can drive the listener to want to find some kind of solution to fix the problem. When this happens in a group, one useful intervention is to ask whether the distressed member is getting what he or she needs from the group right now. This type of intervention can open the door to helping the member express her deeper feelings.

In this session, the group leader commented that Meredith probably doesn't need solutions (which was primarily what she was getting from the group) but needs to grieve. Another member quickly objected and said that Meredith needs to reconstitute. This again is another expression of the difficulty members can have in allowing the expression of difficult emotions. Meredith responded that the losses are hitting her hard—a direct response to the group leader's comment—suggesting that the leader was right on target. Meredith then brought up another loss, her inability to have children.

Meredith's responses to the leader suggest that she felt understood by the leader's comment that she needs to grieve. Given that she needed to grieve and that instead she had been bombarded with advice about how to cope, it would have been useful to check in with her to see if she had felt understood and supported by the group and whether what they had given her had felt helpful.

Facilitating Active Coping.   Having provided an illustration of when focusing on active coping is premature, let us turn to when active coping should be the focus. In those situations patients are encouraged to approach problems in their lives with the assumption that there is something they can do to improve the situation. This general orientation covers all situations including those about which there seems to be very little one can do. With issues such as facing the possibility of a premature death, patients are encouraged to break the problem down into manageable pieces. For some pieces, they may discover that the best way to cope is to express their feelings about it to others. For other pieces, they may realize that there are courses of action they can take to alleviate some of the concern. For instance, if part of the worry is about not being there to watch over and guide their children, they may decide to write letters to their children for them to read when they are older. Whatever the problem, patients are taught to identify the courses of action they can take to better cope with the situation. In some cases this may simply involve learning acceptance. The following example occurred in a brief group for primary breast cancer patients.

The group leader turned to Vivian, who had been quiet, and asked what was going on with her today. Vivian responded that she was feeling tired and hoped her energy would come back. She complained that she felt tired all the time. The group leader asked if she had talked to her doctor about her fatigue. Vivian pointed to her head, saying, "It's all in my head." "Is this something that your doctor said?" he asked. "No," she replied. "This is how I feel about it." Vivian went on to say that she wished she could get some amphetamines to help with her energy. She also stated that when she sleeps she escapes and that last night she found a lump under her breast. She continued, somewhat humorously, "That put me to sleep" and then "Please, dear lord, no more."

These were powerful statements that revealed a good deal about Vivian. Her sleeping to escape and her desire for amphetamines revealed her use of avoidance as a coping strategy. Her use of humor was also a way for her to distance herself from her feelings. Clearly, having discovered a lump under her breast had raised a lot of anxiety in Vivian. This fact was not lost on the group.

The group members quickly responded to the news of the lump by asking Vivian if she had called her doctor. Vivian responded that she had made an appointment to see her doctor in two weeks and that she had no desire to go sooner. "No more doctors," she proclaimed.

These were all provocative statements suggesting that Vivian was in significant distress and that she needed help both to face her feelings and to implement more adaptive coping strategies.

The group leader made the first attempt at helping Vivian access what she was feeling. He asked, "Is finding this lump what's bothering you?" Vivian responded that she didn't know. The leader continued to ask probing questions in an effort to help Vivian access her feelings. She continued to respond with flippant comments, suggesting that not only was she was deeply troubled by the situation but that she was working hard to defend herself from her feelings.

Realizing that another strategy was needed, the co-leader shifted the focus to the group and asked if others had ever had similar feelings. Marilyn said that she can understand how hard it is to face finding a lump. She spoke with emotion about what it was like when she discovered her lump and the emotional roller-coaster she went through as she waited to be tested and then waited for the results. Another member, Betty, also talked about the time that she found a lump. The co-leader asked Betty if she could imagine waiting two weeks not knowing if it was cancer. Betty replied no and described going into the doctor's office and throwing a "hissy fit" because they were planning to do the surgery in three days and not immediately.

This general strategy of pulling in the group members and nudging them in directions in which you want the group to go is an effective way of facilitating supportive interaction. Furthermore, there is much less resistance hearing suggestions from the group members than it is hearing them from the leaders.

With continued probing from the group leaders and the encouragement of the group members, Vivian finally admitted that she was afraid about what she might learn when she goes to the doctor. In the end, Vivian acquiesced and said that she would call her doctor the next day.

This example illustrates the importance of focusing on active coping. However, as crucial as it was to focus on active coping, it was first necessary to help the patient access her internal response to her situation. Her natural way of coping was to use avoidance and humor to protect herself from her terrifying feelings. This also had the unfortunate consequence of keeping her from being proactive about dealing with her disease. Therefore, prior to helping her to change her coping strategies and to adopt one that was more proactive, it was necessary to help her to face the feelings she was trying to avoid. This example also illustrates the vital role that group support plays. Having other group members talk about their own emotional response to similar situations as well as hearing about their active coping strategies enabled Vivian to face her own situation at an emotional level as well as considering more adaptive ways of handling the situation.

RELAXATION AND GUIDED IMAGERY

In our cancer groups the therapists encourage and often rehearse ways of making changes within the group with the hope that similar changes will be possible outside of the group. One technique we use to facilitate this process is self-hypnosis. Hypnosis is a simple shift in the focus of attention that can be used to help patients relax, to manage pain, and to consolidate what has been learned in the group. In this chapter we discuss how it can be used to help patients examine issues that emerge in the group session (Spiegel and Spiegel, 1978). In Chapter 11 we discuss how it can be used to manage pain. Self-hypnosis provides patients with the opportunity to appreciate their current situation, set realistic goals that would improve their quality of life, and construct ways to make this transition within the context of their lives.

We conduct the hypnotic exercise at the end of each meeting and, after several guided self-hypnosis sessions, the patients can begin to use the method at home on their own. Generally, the therapist leads the group through the hypnotic exercise by pulling out a specific theme that is appropriate to each session and when appropriate focusing on pain management. Identifying a theme of the group and using this theme in the self-hypnosis exercise at the end of the meeting is a useful way of helping group members consolidate what has been learned in the session. The induction is approximately five minutes in length, and usually leaves the patients with a sense of restfulness and completion. In addition, patients are left with the feeling of being a collaborator in their own treatment and of having some control.

A simple self-hypnosis induction involves the following:

1. **Induction into self-hypnosis:** The first step is to help the members enter a safe and comfortable state where they are floating comfortably, free of tension and pain.

   Get as comfortable as possible with your arms resting on the arms of your chair. Look up, slowly close your eyes, take a deep breath, let your eyes relax. Imagine a feeling of floating, floating right down through the chair. . . . There will be something pleasant and welcome about this sensation of floating. Each breath you take is deeper and easier. No matter what else might be going on, you can continue to concentrate on this pleasant feeling. Imagine that you are floating in a bath, a lake, a hot tub, or just floating in space.

2. **Pain control:** If any members are experiencing pain, members are instructed to imagine a competing sensation so that the focus is taken

off the pain and put on a sensation that is more tolerable (see Chapter 11 for a discussion of how to work with pain).

If you feel any discomfort now, imagine that this part of your body is becoming warmer or cooler, lighter or heavier, or starting to tingle. Notice how you can place a protective filter of a warm or cool tingling numbness between you and the pain. That's right, just filter the hurt out of the pain. Imagine rubbing snow on the part of your body that hurts or taking a nice warm bath. Filter the hurt out of the pain.

3. **Imagine a screen off in the distance and picture a pleasant scene:** Members are instructed to visualize a screen on which they can place images. This screen can be manipulated in their minds as they wish to help them view whatever image they place there, as will be illustrated later in the exercise.

As you continue to float, you can continue to concentrate effortlessly on that pleasant floating feeling. At the same time, while you imagine yourself floating, in your mind's eye visualize a huge screen. It can be a movie screen, a TV screen, or, if you wish, a piece of clear blue sky. Now imagine something that gives you a lot of pleasure and just let yourself enjoy that image for a minute. . . . Each breath you take is deeper and easier.

4. **The problem screen:** Members are instructed to divide the screen in half and place a problem state on the left side of the screen. The type of problem state is based on the material that emerged in the session. For example, a main theme in the session might be feeling a lack of control about the cancer. During this phase of the exercise, if the image is threatening or difficult to look at, the members can be instructed to manipulate the screen by pushing the screen farther away or making it smaller.

Look up to the screen on the left. Picture on that screen something about the cancer that you can't control. If you find that this image is difficult to look at, make the screen small or push the screen farther away. . . . Each breath you take is deeper and easier.

5. **Return to comfort state:** After holding the picture in their minds for about a minute, members are instructed to return to their comfort state where the body is floating comfortably, unaffected by what is on the screen.

   Now you can let that image go, and focus on the comfortable feeling of your body floating, feeling safe and secure. Each breath you take is deeper and easier.

6. **Right screen is goal state:** Members are instructed to place a goal state or a solution on the right side of the screen—for example, something about the cancer that they can control.

   Now look to the screen on the right. Picture on that screen one thing that you can control about the cancer.

7. **Return to comfort state:** After holding the picture in their minds for about a minute, members are instructed again to return to their comfort state where the body is floating comfortably, unaffected by what is on the screen.

   Now you can let that image go, and focus on the comfortable feeling of your body floating, feeling safe and secure. Each breath you take is deeper and easier.

8. **Look at both screens side by side:** They are now instructed to hold the two images side by side so that they can reflect on both the problem and the solution together and to extract whatever meaning the exercise has had for them.

   Return again to the images on your two screens and hold them side by side. Take a few moments to reflect on what this means to you in a private sense.

9. **Suggestions for future use and bringing them out of the state of self-hypnosis.**

   You can use this exercise as a way to make your body feel more comfortable and as a way of dealing with problems by placing them in a new perspec-

tive. When you are ready, bring yourself out of the state of self-hypnosis by counting backward from 3 to 1. On 3, get ready. On 2, with your eyelids closed, roll up your eyes. On 1 let your eyes open. 3 . . . 2 . . . 1 . . .

In using this split-screen technique, it is important to recognize that the advantage of the technique is that you can tailor what you put on the left and right sides of the screen so that it captures important themes from that particular session. In Table 4.1, we provide some examples of problem-states and solutions that can be placed on the two sides of the screen. Remember that these are intended to be examples only. The possibilities for what you put on the screen are endless. We supply you with these examples only as a way of helping you to think about how to create unique problem and solution states at the end of each session.

TABLE 4.1   Examples of Session Themes for the Split Screen Technique

Problem State	*Goal State*
Picture what someone needs from you.	Picture what you need from that person or from others.
(Following the death of a group member) Picture Mary and the fact that she is gone and will no longer be with us.	Picture something that Mary left with us.
Picture someone you are afraid to get close to for some reason, perhaps for fear of losing them.	Picture that same person from the perspective of the things that drew you to him or her.
Picture one thing that you fear.	Picture one thing that you hope for.
Picture something about which you are anxious.	Picture one thing that you can do about it.
Picture a way in which having cancer isolates you.	Picture something that you have gained because of the cancer.
Picture an aspect of yourself that you once had and is now gone.	Picture an aspect of yourself that remains.
Picture one way in which having cancer has had a negative effect on your relationship with your family.	Picture one way in which having cancer has enhanced your relationship with your family.

SUGGESTIONS FOR
THE FINAL SESSIONS

How and when to terminate supportive-expressive groups is a complex question, particularly when you are working with patients who have advanced disease. This is a question we urge group leaders to consider *before* they start their group. In leading a group for advanced disease, you are dealing with patients who have an illness for which they will need support in one way or another until the day they die. Consequently, it is important to be clear at the outset regarding the length of time the group will be offered and to consider how you will facilitate group members getting the support they need after the group is over.

TERMINATION OF LONG-TERM GROUPS

We have had the unique experience of leading supportive-expressive groups for metastatic breast cancer patients that have continued for as long as eight years. We have added new patients as others died or left, but some members have been with the group since the beginning. This in itself is striking—they gain something from the contact with one another that seems to provide enduring value to them. It is not merely a matter of learning something and moving on. Rather, many group members find the ongoing regular contact is of continuing value. Many have helped others through the final phases of their lives, and hope to maintain the community of support when their time comes. Others find comfort in the ongoing life of the group, as though they will live on in the memory of others in the group, as those who have died continue to do.

Nonetheless, even long-term groups must end sometime. The end of a group is a kind of death, and must be treated with forethought and working through of feelings related to it. It helps to plan the termination well in advance, so members have time to address their feelings and concerns.

Often there is anger. Group members may feel abandoned by the therapists. They may feel it as a withdrawal of concern. To the extent that they have been comforted by one another's presence, they face the threat of having that taken away. At the same time, members may be reluctant to bring up such emotions, fearing that they may drive away the therapists and what remains of their group.

When the termination of one long-term metastatic breast cancer group was discussed, the first reaction was anger: "How can you abandon us like this?" "I don't remember being told we were only promised a year of group." "You can't get people emotionally involved like this and then just end it!" Following the expression of anger was sorrow that the group might end. Members expressed how important the group had been to them, that the group had become a lifeline, that they had grown to love one another. On the heels of acknowledging their sorrow came fear. "Where will I go if my cancer progresses?" "I'm afraid that the group is what keeps me alive." Pain at facing the loss of the group was another reaction. "This is precisely why I was reluctant to join the group in the first place. I knew I would get emotionally attached and that it would hurt to lose people." Other emotions included gratitude for having the opportunity to participate in such a group for so long. Many members also felt that they had "been there" for others who had died, and they wanted understandably to feel that the group would be there for them when their turn came.

Clearly there is grieving to be done at such a time. It involves the therapists helping the group to take stock of their experience: "What will you miss most about the group?" "What will stay with you even after the group is over?" Questions like these can help group members come to terms with the end of the group. After this, many groups enter an active coping phase. This may involve plans to seek support elsewhere, or to continue contact in some different form. In an ordinary group, this would be considered denial and undermining of the necessary grief work. While that could be the case, it may also be a necessary outcome. Groups like this take energy to start, but, like Newton's first law of motion, "An object at rest tends to remain at rest; an object in motion tends to remain in motion," once a group gets started, it wants to continue. There is conservation of momentum. Once they have begun, they often find ways to carry on. Sometimes this involves finding new resources, sometimes meeting monthly in someone's living room, sometimes keeping in touch by phone.

Therefore, when considering ending your involvement in a long-term group, there are several issues to consider. At the outset of the group and whenever a new person joins the group, you should state what your plan is for the length of the group and how much advance warning you will give for its ending. One approach is to make year-long contracts so that once a year you and your group decide whether or not to renew the commitment. If you plan to end the group, it is important to provide a minimum of one month's warning per each year that the group has been in existence, longer if possible. So, if the group has been going for three years, let them know at least three months ahead of time of when you plan to end the group. Remember, this is a minimum. The more advance warning you can give them the better. Thus, if you know at the outset when the group is going to end, tell them. If you simply plan on ending your involvement in the group, it may be possible to bring in a new group leader. This option should be thoroughly discussed with the group members before enacting such a decision. Another option is to have the group disband and to help individual members form another group or join an existing group. All options should be considered and discussed with your group members prior to the end of the group.

Our experience with long-term groups for advanced-stage cancer patients has clearly demonstrated the value of these groups. These groups offer an invaluable and rare resource to these patients. Conducting such groups, however, is a major commitment, not to be taken lightly. Therefore, if you plan to conduct such groups we urge you to consider not only how you will begin them but also how you will eventually bring them to an end.

TERMINATION OF SHORT-TERM GROUPS

If you are planning to lead a group for primary stage disease, then it is both reasonable and sensible to offer a brief and time-limited group because this is what most patients with early-stage disease are seeking. Throughout the course of these sessions, the therapists should occasionally remind the group about the number of sessions remaining. However, we recommend that after approximately two-thirds of the sessions have occurred, the topic of termination should be put on the table as a central issue. At this time, the group should be reminded of the termination date and asked to reflect on their thoughts and feelings about the impending end. It is not uncommon for the group to ask why the sessions have to end or whether it is possible to continue in some way. Although this issue should be addressed directly, it can often deflect attention from the real concern, termination.

The main goal in raising the topic of termination at this time is to bring the issue to the forefront so that group members will begin to reflect on it. This topic is important because ending therapy raises issues for everyone: For cancer patients it is likely to raise issues that are relevant to living with a potentially life-threatening illness.

FINAL SESSIONS

There are bound to be many feelings activated by thoughts of termination, particularly if members have evolved into a close and cohesive group. Termination raises issues of direct relevance to their cancer concerns, particularly grieving losses and having to get on with their lives in spite of these losses. There will be feelings about losing the close, supportive network they have established and fears about having to make it on their own. Similarly, it will reactivate feelings of being alone. There may be anger at being abandoned in a time of need. Some members may appear to feel very little about the therapy coming to an end. This may be a defensive response to protect themselves from feelings of vulnerability and dependence on others for support; it may also be a genuine reaction to termination. No matter what kinds of responses individuals have to the impending termination date, it is important to address and explore them fully. The members are encouraged to bring all their thoughts, feelings, and concerns about the matter to the group.

An important consequence of exploring feelings evoked by termination is that it is an opportunity for the group members to say directly what they have meant to each other. The sense of connection and understanding they have received from each other is a precious and unique gift about which they will have heartfelt feelings. For these same reasons, the end of the group presents a tremendous loss. It also symbolizes losses they have previously experienced and may experience in the future. Consequently, termination presents an opportunity to work through one set of losses and in so doing can prepare them to deal with losses that lie ahead.

The last couple of sessions are a time for the group to consolidate what has been gained over the course of treatment. The leaders can help the members reflect on how far they have come since entering the group. Where are they now with the issues they came in with? Has anything changed for them and in what way? Where had they hoped they would be at this point in the treatment? Are they feeling as alone with their illness? What have they learned about themselves and how might this be helpful to them in dealing with the cancer? What changes have they made or decided to make in their lives? What have they found to be especially helpful in the group? The leaders can take an active role in highlighting the advances each member has made.

Another important question to address is whether any important issues have been avoided. Are there any concerns that they would have liked to address but didn't? If there are such issues that they identify, there may still be time to work on them. For issues that the members have actively and consistently avoided, the goal is to have the members at least recognize that these issues exist, even though they are not yet ready to deal with them.

Termination presents an opportunity to deal directly with issues that have symbolic relevance—death and loss, one's essential aloneness, taking stock of where one has come and wants to go from here. Because these issues are difficult, however, there is often a tendency to avoid them. As termination looms, discussion frequently turns to how the group can be made to continue. Sometimes this takes the form of discussing how to meet independently without the group leaders. Some groups will even arrange to hire another therapist. These attempts to make the group continue are a powerful statement about the importance of the group to the members. Therapists can use this to help the group openly acknowledge its importance. Some members will decide that this particular experience was sufficient and that they are ready to go on with their lives. The positive message and validity behind this position should also be affirmed.

However, as the group comes to an end, each member must also confront her own feelings about saying good-bye, about the death of the group, about the loss of something important. She must face again her existential aloneness, having to move forward without the assurance of the group being there to turn to. Chances are that she will have made significant ties with various members in the group, which will undoubtedly continue. Nevertheless, the group itself will no longer be there for her. It is time for her to take stock of where she has come, of the resources she has available to her, and to decide how she wants to proceed into the future. She must grieve what she leaves behind, yet at the same time take with her into the future all of the support, hope, and self-renewal she has gained.

WORKING WITH A CO-LEADER

SELECTION OF GROUP LEADERS

When we have put groups together, our preference has been to have two leaders facilitate the groups. There are several advantages to this. One is that it enables us to find two individuals who between them have a broad range of relevant experience. Our ideal group leaders are individuals with experience in conducting group therapy, knowledge of the illness, and experience in working with this population.

In an effort to achieve our ideal, we have put together co-leader teams of oncology nurses and psychotherapists. This has worked reasonably well, although there are some pitfalls to be aware of. One of these is that if the oncology nurse has no background in group psychotherapy, he or she is prone to falling into the "information-giver" role. There is also a tendency for the group members to push the oncology nurse into that role. Consequently, when using oncology nurses it is important to provide training prior to the start of the group as well as ongoing supervision. When these teams work well, they are usually excellent. This is because there is one person who has the ability to understand what the patient is going through and therefore is alert to issues that need to be addressed. The other person has the skills to facilitate the kind of exploration and mutual support that is needed to negotiate the issues.

We have also successfully used co-leader teams of psychotherapists where one of the co-leaders herself has had cancer. This has a similar advantage to the nurse/psychotherapist team. The potential pitfall here is that the co-leader who has had cancer can be prone to losing her therapeutic distance because the issues can strike so close to home. Here again it is important for the co-leaders to have ongoing supervision as well as an open and trusting relationship with each other.

We have successfully used co-leader teams of psychotherapists who have no personal experience with or training in oncology. In these cases, it is useful to try to team up a psychotherapist who has no experience with the population with a psychotherapist who has had some experience. It is not a good idea to have two people co-leading a group with no prior knowledge of cancer or experience with the population.

Groups led by one group leader are another option, although one that we avoid if we can. Certainly, for practical and financial reasons it is not always possible to do so. There are several advantages to two co-leaders. The primary advantage is that when two therapists work together, one can be directly involved in the group process while the other can be sitting back and observing the group process at another level. For example, one therapist might be helping a member explore some important issues. While this is going on, the other therapist can be scanning the group to observe the reactions of the other members. The information that the observing therapist is gathering can then be brought into the group either to deepen the exploration or to bring other group members into the discussion. When there is only one group leader, it is clearly much more difficult to be working at both levels simultaneously. A second advantage to two group leaders is that if one leader is absent due to illness or vacation, the group can still meet with the remaining group leader. Having stated why we prefer two co-leaders, we also want to be clear that we do lead groups with only one leader when we need to. Certainly it is better to have a group with one leader than to have no leader at all.

GROUND RULES FOR WORKING IN GROUP

A few ground rules about working together in the group will greatly enhance your working relationship. One important rule to adhere to is that whenever your co-leader makes an intervention, give the group members time to respond. Do not immediately follow up your co-leader's intervention with a different intervention. This has the effect of nullifying the first intervention. If the group has not responded to an important intervention your co-leader has made, then you should step in and follow up that intervention with one that reinforces it. When you and your co-leader are working in concert, you can build upon each other's intervention to maximize the impact of your work together.

Another strategy for working well together is to share the responsibilities in leading the group. The ideal co-leading team is one where both leaders are viewed as equal and vital to the group process. At a superficial level, this attitude can be conveyed by sharing the housekeeping tasks such as setting up the room or contacting group members who have been absent. You may be surprised to find how small tasks can take on great significance not only for the group members but the leaders as well.

As in any form of therapy, therapists should be aware of their own emotional response to issues that emerge in the group. Emotional responses to the group process are natural. Because the incidence of cancer is high and people often want to work in areas in which they have a personal interest, a significant percentage of the leaders will themselves have had cancer. If a leader is a cancer patient, he or she should be especially attuned to his or her own emotional response to issues raised in group so that it does not impede the group process. Being a cancer survivor can be an asset if the group leader is able to be clear about his or her own experience and bring what he or she has learned and struggled with to the group. However, the leaders must also be careful that their own fears and anxieties do not prevent them from helping the group broach frightening topics. Any anxieties that arise for each of them during the group should be shared with their co-leader afterwards so that the co-leader will be attuned to areas where she or he may need to shoulder more of the therapeutic responsibility.

A successful group depends on a healthy match between the leaders. To this end, it is important that the co-leaders know beforehand that they are of like mind as to the purpose of the group and the basic therapeutic approach. Each leader will have her or his own strengths and weaknesses. The best co-leaders will recognize these and work to build on each other's strengths and to offset each other's weaknesses.

GIVING FEEDBACK TO EACH OTHER

To a large extent, a positive group experience depends on how well group leaders work together. A critical factor for a successful co-leading relationship is that the co-leaders be open with and supportive of each other. Thus, our main advice is for group leaders to try to be as open and candid with each other as possible. Following each group meeting, the leaders should spend time reviewing what has transpired. This is an opportunity to review what has gone well, address concerns you might have about particular group members, plan for the next group, and to discuss how the two of you are working together. One method that we have found to be invaluable is to review videotapes of your sessions with your co-leader. This provides a much more objective perspective and enables you to see what you actually did or, more important, what you could have done.

How to Provide Feedback.   One of the more important tasks in which you should engage when rehashing a group is to provide feedback to each other. This will greatly enhance how you work together and will exponentially increase your learning experience. If there are disagreements about how to lead the group, it is essential that these be aired outside of group and that a compromise be reached. Remember, however, that giving and receiving feedback can feel threatening. In fact, expect to feel threatened. This is a normal response.

We suggest a number of guidelines for giving and receiving feedback, to make the experience as constructive and nonthreatening as possible. First, think about the feedback you want to give. Are you trying to be helpful to your co-leader or is it something that would be helpful for you? If it is something to help you, share this so that the receiver will better understand what you are saying. Is it something that you or your co-leader will be able to do anything about? Give the feedback in a descriptive, not interpretive, manner. State your feelings about what happened, rather than drawing conclusions. Try not to overload your co-leader by stating everything you have to say all at once. Give the feedback in manageable chunks, preferably taking turns with your co-leader. Finally, don't forget to give each other feedback about what you liked about each other's interventions and what went well.

How to Receive Feedback.   Receiving feedback is just as challenging as giving it. Listen to what has been said and restate it so that you are clear that you heard it correctly. Give yourself a minute to reflect on what has been said. Do you understand it? Try to be aware of your own feelings about the feedback, as they can sometimes get in the way of listening and learning. When responding to the feedback, address the issue, but also remember to share your reactions to the feedback itself. The person giving the feedback needs to know your reactions so that he or she will not go away concerned about how you felt. You may even want to give your co-leader feedback on how he or she gives feedback.

In co-leading a group with someone there will inevitably be issues that arise between the group leaders. Our advice is to work toward addressing and resolving these issues just as you strive to help your patients work through their own tough issues. A good working relationship between you and your co-leader will be important for making your group a positive experience for everyone involved.

CONCLUSION

These treatment strategies are designed to help you help your patients live fully in the moment and in the time they have left. This is accomplished by helping them address and express their concerns openly and honestly. Exploring all emotional states and thoughts pertaining to their cancer gives the important message that no thought or feeling is too frightening to face. Furthermore, it can be immeasurably validating to discover that negative feelings and disturbing thoughts are shared by others. Through open and honest sharing of feelings, concerns, thoughts, and ideas with others in a safe and supportive environment, patients come to recognize that they are not alone and in fact have a forum in which to express their full experience. Working in the here-and-now provides opportunities for patients to address their issues directly, thereby providing greater opportunity for growth. Learning active coping strategies to handle their problems provides patients with powerful tools for living with cancer. Relaxation exercises are one such active coping strategy that they can take from the group experience and apply in their everyday lives. Using the tools we have provided in this chapter in the context of a good working relationship with your co-leader will set the stage for a successful group experience.

CHAPTER 5

Building Group Support

A support group is often the only place where patients feel understood, accepted, and a little less alone (Spiegel et al., 1981). The common bond of having a shared problem very rapidly creates an uncommon sense of belonging. The very thing that excludes members from a sense of belonging in the world of the well is their ticket of admission to the group. The shared experience in living with the disease means that frequently little needs to be said in order to communicate what is going on for them. As the group matures, and bonds and trust develop, patients come to know that the group will be there to support and understand them; and when the group ends, these friendships frequently continue. Thus, simply by being in a group, patients often vastly improve the social support they receive.

Although supportive behaviors develop naturally in a cancer support group, the group leaders play an important role in the early stages of a group and at critical moments in the life of the group. Before describing a variety of situations where interventions from the group leaders are essential, we give an example of a group interaction where the group members naturally and freely gave much needed support to a group member.

SUPPORT THAT OCCURS NATURALLY

In an established group there is often little the leader needs to do to facilitate supportive interactions. This example occurred in a long-term group of metastatic breast cancer patients.

One of the members, Anne, struggled more than most, partly because her cancer was re-lentlessly progressing and partly because of many other traumas she had experienced throughout her life. Anne was terrified that she was running out of time and felt that she had tried all that conventional medicine had to offer. She had learned about an al-ternative diet that involved eating only raw foods, drinking wheatgrass, and having en-emas twice daily. She had recently returned from a retreat for followers of this diet.

Anne returned to group after an extended absence looking frail and jaundiced. She had been on the diet for two months and to everyone's horror had shed 30 pounds from her tiny body. A couple of weeks after her return, Anne told the group that she had a rapidly growing tumor in her breast and had decided to change her diet and resume chemotherapy. She thanked everyone for the cards she received during the week that urged her to "Eat!" Although she was trying to eat, she struggled with eating anything other than raw foods, as her body no longer seemed to tolerate anything cooked. Thus, she was grateful to a friend who brought her a large pot of chicken broth, which she was pleased to find she could digest. The group was relieved to hear that she was at last open to eating other foods and encouraged her to continue trying.

After an animated discussion about how the members felt about their lack of control over the disease, Anne volunteered that she felt guilty. "What are you feeling guilty about?" one of the leaders asked. "I didn't follow the diet well enough. I was only giv-ing myself an enema once every two days when I should have been doing it twice a day. Maybe it's my fault that the tumor is growing."

The group quickly rallied to dissuade Anne of her self-blame. "Don't feel guilty," they urged her, almost pleading with her. It was clearly painful for these women to see Anne, who had already suffered so much, be so harsh with herself. In their efforts to talk her out of her guilt, one woman focused on the fact that the people who were advocating this diet were healthy and that it wasn't appropriate to compare herself to them. The next woman said angrily that she resented that our culture tells us that we are respon-sible for this disease. "I agree," replied another. "I was told that if I hadn't had the stress of building my house the year before my diagnosis, I wouldn't have developed cancer." One woman said gently, "Anne, I feel bad that at a time when you have the burden of chemotherapy, you also have the burden of feeling responsible for your disease progress-ing." "When you should be loving yourself instead," responded another. "You didn't do anything wrong. You didn't do anything to deserve this."

The love and concern that was in the room was palpable, and although the support may not have undone the effect of years of struggling with the tragedies that had un-folded in Anne's life, Anne appeared less burdened and a little lighter of spirit that evening when she left the room.

FACILITATING SUPPORTIVE
INTERACTIONS

As the preceding example illustrates, support from group members can naturally emerge. However, this is not always the case, which is particularly true early on in the life of a group when the members are first learning what it means to be in a support group. This is a time for the leaders to model support. Leaders must do this by showing interest in each patient's story, expressing empathy for difficult situations, or asking about a patient's emotional reactions to what has been described. It must be conveyed that everyone's experience is important and of interest. Everyone has something to contribute.

There are still other times when the therapist must play an active role in eliciting support from the group, such as when a patient seems particularly alienated.

Marsha, for example, was a young woman with early-stage breast cancer and was fortunate in requiring only surgery to remove the malignant lump. While she recognized how fortunate she was, she also found that her particular situation made her feel alienated both inside and outside the group. In her daily life, she found that no one seemed to understand how concerned and preoccupied she was with having been diagnosed with cancer. Everyone thought that because the lump had been removed, she had nothing more to fear. This was not how she experienced it, however. She was afraid. She found herself ruminating about the possibility that her cancer might return.

In the group Marsha felt different. Everyone else seemed to have more serious problems because of the more advanced stages of their illnesses. She felt that they could not understand why she was so fearful about her situation. In one meeting Marsha complained at length about not feeling understood by her husband and her friends. "Other people have their own problems. They don't want to hear about mine," she said. "How can we be helpful to you?" asked one of the leaders.

In response to this question, Marsha tried to convey her sense that she is in a different situation from the rest of the group. "Your problems aren't like mine," she said. "Mine are more involved. They are . . . Well, for you it's just your cancer. For me it's . . . I don't know . . . It's . . . I'm rambling here." The more she spoke, the more inarticulate and distant she became. Finally, she said, "Oh, forget it. Let someone else talk."

Although the leader had tried to support Marsha by asking how the group could be helpful, Marsha was feeling too alienated to be able to ask anything of the group. At this point, it was as though Marsha was drifting further and further away. Somehow she needed to be reached. At the same time, she was beginning to feel uncomfortable being the focus of the group and needed to be taken off the hot seat. It was time to shift the focus to others and at the same time counter Marsha's feeling of alienation. Accordingly, the leader asked the group if they had any reactions to what Marsha had been saying.

This intervention was an invitation to the group to provide their perspective on what they had heard, thereby enabling individual members to spontaneously and genuinely give their support and understanding. It was helpful for Marsha to hear that the other members did not agree that she was different from the rest of them. She too had to cope with the uncertainty and fear that the cancer would recur, they argued. The discussion that ensued was helpful in reducing Marsha's sense of alienation.

HANDLING A PROBLEMATIC
EXPRESSION OF SUPPORT

The situation with Marsha provides a good example of when leaders must play an active role in eliciting support. The responsiveness of the group members to a request that they provide support to members in need is what you can expect most often from your groups. Occasionally, however, situations will arise when the group or individual members do not respond in the most desirable fashion even though they may be trying to be supportive. When this happens, the leaders again must play an active role. Such a situation, referred to briefly in Chapter 3, occurred in one of our primary breast cancer groups.

One of the members, Melanie, had recently been diagnosed with metastatic breast cancer. Prior to returning to group, she contacted one of the leaders to discuss her situation and to find out if she was still welcome in the group. The leader reassured her that her status as a group member was in no way altered because of her metastasis. Melanie and the leader talked about how they should handle the situation and the possible effect her news would have on the group. The leader warned Melanie that it would likely raise the anxiety of all the group members regarding their own health but that Melanie should not feel responsible for the group's anxiety. Her metastasis does not alter their individual situations and the anxiety they have about recurrence exists regardless of her situation. Melanie was reassured to hear this but also felt that she wanted to ask the group for herself about whether they would want her to remain in the group.

At the next meeting, Melanie told the group her devastating news. She was tearful as she explained her situation and the group sat in stunned silence. Melanie then raised the question about whether she should remain in the group given that it had begun as a primary breast cancer group. "Of course I want to stay because I need all the support I can get. Nevertheless," she went on, "the group is here for the majority, not the minority, and so I will have every understanding if you decide that I should find another group." Cynthia, who was seated next to her, took her hand and said, "Of course, we want to be with you during this. It breaks my heart to hear that this has happened. How could we ever abandon you or anyone else in the group when something like this happens." Certainly, Cynthia's response was just what Melanie needed to hear. However, this was a question for all members, and so each woman felt obliged to respond.

The next woman to speak was Loretta. Loretta had psychological problems as well as breast cancer. She coped by being overly intellectualized and detached from her emotional experience. Loretta had been in another breast cancer group where a similar situation had arisen, and so it was the experience of that group that Loretta referred to as she tried in her way to be supportive. Loretta spoke at length in a distant and abstract manner and the shift in the emotional tone of the group was striking and uncomfortable. One member who was sitting beside Loretta moved an empty chair out of the circle and her own chair farther from Loretta, as though to distance herself emotionally as well as physically from Loretta. "Let me tell you the story of that group," Loretta said. "They decided to let that member stay, and even though she did die, it turned out okay that she had stayed."

There was silence following Loretta's speech. It seemed that no one knew what to say.

This was a critical moment in the group for two reasons. One was the concern for Melanie and how she was feeling about Loretta's feedback. The other was that Loretta ran the risk of alienating herself from the group by her deviant response. This was a moment where an intervention by one of the leaders was essential.

In intervening in such a situation, it is useful to consider what Loretta was trying to do as well as how she did it. It appeared that the basic message Loretta wanted to convey was that Melanie should remain in the group. The way she communicated this, however, was to tell a story about somebody else. In so doing, she failed to talk about her own feelings about whether she wanted Melanie to remain in the group. With this in mind, the goal was to help Loretta speak directly to Melanie about her feelings.

The therapist turned to Loretta and said, "Loretta, what is the message you are wanting to convey to Melanie with this story?"

That question enabled Loretta to speak directly about her feelings for Melanie and to provide the kind of support that was needed.

Helping Loretta speak directly to Melanie was important for both Loretta and Melanie as well as the rest of the group. It was important for Melanie because she needed a direct answer to whether or not Loretta wanted her to remain in the group. It was important for the other group members because it helped them to see what Loretta was really trying to say, perhaps giving them a little empathy regarding her difficulty in speaking plainly and directly about what she feels. They could see that although she sounded deviant, she in fact was no different from anyone else in her desire to support Melanie. Finally, it was important for Loretta because it was a small lesson in learning how to speak directly. More importantly, however, it also prevented her from being ostracized or scapegoated by the group.

IDENTIFYING MISSED OPPORTUNITIES
FOR MUTUAL SUPPORT

There are other types of situations where members may intend to be supportive of each other but fail to do so, thereby requiring the leader to intervene. For example, when a member brings up a topic that is difficult for her, it is often the case that the topic is difficult for other group members as well. In these cases it is not unusual to find one or more members shift the topic to something easier. It is also not unusual for the person or even the entire group to be aware that this shift has occurred. The leaders must again play an active role to return the focus to where it should be. This is important both for the patient who has raised the issue and for those who find the subject uncomfortable.

Such was the case when Melanie brought up the fact that she was at a high risk for recurrence. (This was prior to learning that her cancer had metastasized.) The group had been talking about the anxiety of making treatment decisions, such as whether to have chemotherapy as well as radiation therapy. Melanie stated that she did not want to second-guess the decisions she had made. "I'm at an 85 percent risk for recurrence. That's too bloody high as far as I'm concerned. I don't want to think about whether I should have done something different." Mary responded, "Trina's in a different position, isn't she, be-

cause she has a third breast." Suddenly the topic shifted to whether Trina had stated that she had a third breast under her arm. This abrupt and baffling shift of topic catapulted the group into an animated discussion of whether some women have third breasts.

The anxiety that was stimulated by Melanie's statement about being at a high risk of recurrence was clearly more than the group could tolerate. Suddenly, the peculiarity of Trina's third breast was a much more compelling topic than Melanie's concern. It is important to return the focus of the discussion to the material that stimulated the anxiety both for the sake of Melanie and for the members themselves. The aim here is twofold: One is to give Melanie the support she needs. The other is to help the group members voice and work through the fears that are underlying their anxiety-driven response. Thus, the leader might respond with "I'm wondering how each of you felt hearing that Melanie is at an 85 percent chance of recurrence?" Notice that it is not necessary to comment on the subject of Trina's third breast. Often it is better simply to ignore the change of subject and shift the focus back to where it had been, although it is sometimes useful to acknowledge the other topic and move on.

MANAGING DISAGREEMENTS

Members frequently fail to be supportive when they disagree with the behavior or decisions of another member. Often, this disagreement is stimulated by anxiety such as when a patient is critical about the treatment decisions made by another member, especially when someone decides to turn to alternative medicine or to give up treatment altogether. In fact, the group leaders themselves may be dismayed at the decisions of the patient. Nevertheless, it does no one any good to criticize the patient for his or her decision. Rather it is a time to elicit as much understanding as possible about the patient's unique situation and point of view.

It is helpful to assume that the behavior or decision makes sense within the context of the patient's experience. Thus, the goal is to help the patient to share her experience with the group so that it can be understood. Usually this is all that is required to facilitate the support of other members. They still might not agree with the patient's decisions but they understand why it has been made.

Sometimes it is necessary to help the critical member examine her criticism to see what may be fueling it. This is especially important when a member seems entrenched in her critical stance. In such cases, underlying the criticism is usually a concern the person has about herself. One way to begin this exploration is to ask the critic what she fears for the patient. Once the fear has been named, the next step is to help the critic examine whether the fear has any personal relevance.

> Brenda was a single woman who had been diagnosed with metastatic breast cancer. Upon joining our support group, she quickly became attached to Anne, an older woman, who, in addition to having an aggressive cancer, had suffered many traumas throughout her life and as a result had learned to rely upon herself. Brenda appreciated the indomitable strength of Anne and, at the same time, was painfully aware of her vulnerability. When Anne became deathly ill, Brenda desperately wanted to be helpful to her. She offered to run errands, buy her groceries, take her to doctor's appointments, or simply drop by to visit. Anne refused it all.
>
> When Brenda described to the group her unsuccessful attempts to help Anne, she sounded increasingly more critical of Anne's refusal to accept help. "What are you concerned about?" the group leader asked. "I'm worried about Anne being left alone to die," Brenda replied. Although this concern about Anne was reasonable, there seemed to be more at stake here. The therapist continued to probe. "Brenda, it seems as though there is more to this than just your concern for Anne. Like Anne, you also live alone. Does this concern relate to you in any way?" Brenda hesitated. "Yes," she admitted. "That's my biggest fear—dying alone."

Recognizing this response as an opportunity to address Brenda's own propensity to refuse help, the therapist asked her how the group could be helpful to her. The ensuing discussion was one of many the group would have about how they could ensure that each of them would not be left to die alone.

BUILDING OUTSIDE SUPPORT AMONG GROUP MEMBERS

In traditional group psychotherapy the aim is to use the group experience as a microcosm of what goes on for patients in their daily lives. In a psychotherapy group, members will recapitulate their experiences and patterns of relating in the outside world. Thus, it is important that the only interaction the group members have with each another is what occurs under the watchful eye of the group leaders and other members. If group members interact outside of group, that material and those patterns of relating become unavailable for processing. The aim of psychotherapy groups is to facilitate change within the individual such as a change in character structure or modifying problematic behavior patterns.

The aim of supportive-expressive psychotherapy groups, however, is not character change but rather to support individuals in living with a life-threatening disease. Thus, unlike the standard psychotherapy group, we actively encourage group members to socialize outside of group. The support that group members give to one another outside of group can be just as important as the support they give to each other in the group. We have found this to be especially true in our long-standing advanced cancer groups. Some of these groups have been meeting for years, and the relationships that have formed extend well beyond the confines of the group room. Phone calls and letters are exchanged, members visit each other, meals are shared, important occasions are celebrated, and those who are ill are cared for. There are even occasions when not only the group members but also the leaders meet with the members outside of group.

Over time some or all group members will develop a desire to meet outside of the group setting. We encourage this while we are also careful not to communicate that it is our expectation that group members have contact outside of group. A desire to extend a relationship beyond the confines of a weekly group meeting is something that must develop naturally. However, because our aim is to enhance support for the group members, we are as facilitating of this as possible, such as by offering to disseminate lists of names and phone numbers to the group members if they wish.

Rachel was the newest member in our metastatic breast cancer group. She was in her early forties and had recently been diagnosed with a very aggressive cancer. During her brief tenure time in our group, Rachel watched Anne struggle as Anne tried every treatment possible to slow down the progression of her disease. Anne's indomitable spirit, in spite of everything she had suffered in her life, was deeply affecting to Rachel. We had not been seeing Anne regularly in group for some time. She was either away to try some alternative treatment or too ill to come to group. When she did come, she inspired everyone with her determination to keep fighting.

During one of Anne's absences, Rachel talked about her desire to spend some time with Anne. She said she fantasized about inviting her to spend a weekend at an ocean-side resort, where they could walk, if Anne was up to it, or just sit by the window watching the waves lap the shore. As Rachel spoke about this she seemed uncertain

about whether she should impose herself upon Anne in this way. The group encouraged
her to do it. Several weeks later, Rachel and Anne made their trek to the ocean. Rachel
smiled as she described their weekend away. We can only guess what this time meant to
her, since as it turned out both Anne and Rachel had little time left. Anne died a few
months later and Rachel a few short weeks after that.

The support that our group members give to each other outside of the group meetings is remarkable. Particularly in long-term groups, the group members can begin to seem like an extended family. Sick members are regularly checked up on, food is lovingly prepared and brought to the sick member's home, members are accompanied to medical appointments, notes are sent back and forth, and weekend excursions are taken.

PROBLEMS THAT CAN ARISE WHEN MEMBERS SOCIALIZE OUTSIDE THE GROUP

Even though we encourage the establishment of relationships among group members outside the group, having members socialize is not without its problems. One of the main reasons is that it is important to be aware of all events that occur between group members. This is necessary in order to have the fullest understanding about what transpires in group. For instance, if there was conflict that occurred outside of group and no one except the members involved were aware of it, then interactions could occur in group that only make sense if one has this knowledge. There might be tension that is felt in the group but the group leaders and other members are unaware of its origin. This can be very detrimental. This type of scenario is not all that common but it can happen. For this reason, we recommend that at the beginning of the group, ground rules are established that include the group members committing to bring back to the group any outside event that they think may have the potential to disrupt the group process.

Even with these precautions, however, problems can arise. It is quite natural for a member to feel more affinity for some people than for others. Consequently, small subgroupings can emerge. This is not necessarily bad. It becomes a problem, though, when it begins to feel to some members either that they are left out or that there is an in-group and an out-group.

The following example was experienced in an HIV-positive group we were conducting. Although this is not a cancer group, the same issues apply. HIV groups are similar to cancer groups in many ways. There are, however, important differences between HIV and cancer groups, which we describe in Chapter 9.

Bob was the newest member of an HIV-positive group. It was a small group consisting of four gay men. Not only was Bob the newest member, he was also the youngest and had only recently been diagnosed as HIV infected. Bob came to the group with a need to talk about his experience and to seek the support of men in similar circumstances. Before entering the group, Bob met with the group leaders for orientation and was informed of the ground rules regarding any socializing outside of group. At the time that Bob entered the group, two of the three group members, Jonathon and Peter, had become friends and during the course of the meetings would occasionally make reference to things that indicated their friendship and the frequency of their contact outside of group. Jonathon was a strong personality. He was a long-term survivor of HIV and a survivor in many other ways. Peter, on the other hand, was newly diagnosed and quiet. Bob and Jonathon somehow never hit it off. Perhaps both Bob and Jonathon were too opinionated for each other. Whatever the case, one day following the group meeting Bob stayed behind to speak to the group leaders. He expressed concern about the friendship of Jonathon and Peter. "Isn't this against the rules?" he asked. As he talked about his feelings, we learned that during meetings when only Jonathon, Peter, and Bob were there, he felt on the outside. Bob began to express anger toward Jonathon for some of his opinions and for overpowering Peter.

This interchange was difficult for a variety of reasons. First, it was occurring outside of group. Ordinarily all important discussions should occur within the group. Second, it appeared that there was a good chance that Bob would decide to leave the group. Third, we were talking about group members who were not present.

We told Bob that we were glad he was bringing this up because it was important to do so if it was troubling him. We explained again the rules regarding socializing with group members outside the group. We then asked him to say more about his feelings on the outside. As he talked about his feelings he acknowledged that they were reminiscent of the feelings he had of being left out as a youngster. He readily admitted that he might be bringing some of this "baggage" into the situation. He realized that what he really wanted was the opportunity to become friends with both Jonathon and Peter. Finally, we urged Bob to bring this issue up in group. We reiterated how important the issue was for the group as a whole and our appreciation that he gave voice to his feelings. Bob left that night with a renewed commitment to the group and the resolve to work through these difficult feelings.

TAKING THE GROUP TO A GROUP MEMBER'S HOME

When a member has become too ill to attend the group meetings, we try to take the group to the ill member's home. Sometimes we have met for weeks on end at the home of an ill member because of the group's desire to have the contact and to support one another.

In one of our metastatic breast cancer groups, our first time at the home of a very ill member was very moving.

Teresa was clearly dying and the change in her was striking. She needed help simply moving on the couch, her color was very poor, and she looked alternately like a little child curled up on the couch with a pillow shaped like a dog bone, and then like an old woman. She spoke weakly and her consciousness was clouded somewhat by the pain medication. She lay on the sofa, often drifting away, yet managing to tell us how much she appreciated the fact that we came. Her strongest concern was reserved for her five-year-old son, who she knew would be taken away from the home by her former husband. We all knew she was dying and that the good-byes we were saying were likely to be the final good-byes. She responded with special emotion to Diane. Diane talked tearfully about her brother dying from cancer and her concern for the three children who were left behind with a mother who seemed more concerned about herself than anyone else. She said, despite that, the children have turned out wonderfully and speak of their father all the time. She said, "Sometimes you just don't know how things will turn out, Teresa." Tears welled in Teresa's eyes as Diane spoke to her. Clearly Teresa and Diane had a special bond.

Sarah spoke emotionally about being scared. Jane said, "I'm next." Nonetheless, they talked about drawing strength from the way that Teresa had handled her illness. The group leader told Teresa that he admired the way she had coped with the continuous adversity in her life and how she had managed to make something beautiful out of it. For the last half hour as Teresa's energy had clearly been spent, the group talked about other issues, such as how other members were. It was a sad but direct meeting in which the members were facing what they feared and yet felt good that they had had the chance to see Teresa one last time. Indeed, Diane commented afterwards that this was the first time they had had such an opportunity just before someone died to visit with them and how good it felt to be able to do that.

ATTENDING A MEMORIAL SERVICE

Funerals and memorial services are some of the most important events in the life of a supportive-expressive group. In one of our long-standing advanced breast cancer groups, Joanne, a beloved but excessively private member, unexpectedly died.

Joanne had been in the group for two years and during that time had become a central group member, valued especially for the wise and thoughtful feedback she could give to others regarding almost any situation. However, Joanne was also notable for how unrevealing she could be.

During Joanne's tenure with the group there had been several deaths and for some reason this group had yet to experience the death of a member who had been willing to be emotionally present with the group until the end. Each of the deaths that had occurred had been of women who were either hiding the reality of the situation from themselves or who had chosen to withdraw from the group and to die alone. This engendered a good deal of pain and regret in the group, and Joanne had on each of these occasions heard the group members bemoan the fact that they had been shut out. The unexpected death of Joanne after an absence of several weeks came as a bitter blow to the group. How could Joanne, after all they had lived through together, shut them out like this? In the end, how well did they even know Joanne?

The memorial service turned out to be very helpful to the group members who attended. Perhaps because they knew how incompletely Joanne shared herself with people in her life, Joanne's family created a memorial service that painted a rich and powerful picture of this remarkable woman. The group learned that there was much they did not know about her. The group had an inkling that Joanne was an accomplished woman, but the full extent of her accomplishments was far beyond what the group realized. Neither did they know that she had lived her childhood haunted by a mysterious and life-threatening illness that was finally diagnosed and remedied when she was seventeen. Perhaps, more importantly, they did not realize the complexity of her personality. Joanne, indeed, was a private person. Even though she was exceedingly confident, beautiful, and intelligent, she was also shy and modest. Over the course of two hours, the group was able to fill in the missing pieces for this much-loved group member. Although it was too late to give Joanne the support that each member had wanted to give, the memorial service presented an opportunity for the remaining group members to support one another. After the service, the members and group leaders gathered together to talk about what the service and Joanne meant to them.

CONCLUSION

Group support is a process that occurs naturally and that can also benefit from the guidance of skilled group leaders. Sometimes the group leaders merely need to step aside to allow the support to be expressed unhindered.

At other times, the group leader may be needed to help members navigate through difficult terrain. Helping patients to find a way to give support in difficult circumstances or to extend their support outside the confines of the group is an important role that the group leaders play. In the setting of providing group support for life-threatening illness, members are crafting a new network of social support, not merely trying out interpersonal techniques for use in the "real" world. The therapists' ability to use the group process to intensify intimacy during the group can reinforce the bonds created among members, which can then extend outside the formal group. Having a serious illness can be stigmatizing and alienating. The sense of belonging that develops in support groups is a powerful antidote to this isolation.

CHAPTER 6

Encouraging Patients to Explore Their Experience and Express Their Emotions

RATIONALE FOR OPEN EXPRESSION

Our years of experience with cancer patients have led us to the conviction that the open expression of emotion of all kinds is therapeutic, even the expression of fear, sadness, anxiety, and anger. Open expression reduces dysphoria, leads to resolution of problems, and counters isolation. This is important since there are multiple powerful roots of the tendency to suppress emotions, especially of the "negative" kind. Many with cancer and other serious illnesses do not want to give in to their feelings about their situation—imagining that they are being strong if they do not admit, even to themselves, that they have feelings about their illness. This is often reinforced by the prevalent belief that having a positive attitude is good for your health, and may even contribute to fighting the disease. Furthermore, outbursts of emotion are generally not welcomed in the medical setting.

The idea that open expression of feeling is a good thing would seem to be contrary to common sense and common practice. Why talk about something sad or threatening if you can't do anything about it anyway? Won't you just discourage yourself by attending to the grimmer aspects of existence? Indeed, some alternative medicine practitioners insist that maintaining a positive attitude, which means a conviction that the incurable will be cured, is essential to recovery. Allowing yourself to give in to depressing thoughts is considered tantamount to yielding to the disease, turning your body over to the cancer, and letting it have its way with you. Furthermore, many fear that giving vent to their sadness or fear will be like opening Pandora's box: Once the crying starts, it will never stop. Ironically, the more one attempts to suppress feeling, the more powerful and uncontrollable it ultimately becomes. This is a lesson well taught in the group setting, where members can witness each other entering and exiting from strong emotional states and can try out an emotional reaction in response to someone else's situation before delving into one of their own.

We have evidence that attempting to put such thoughts out of your mind does not work anyway. For example, we studied 101 women with metastatic breast cancer (Classen, Koopman et al., 1996), giving them measures of mood disturbance and coping. We sought to discover whether emotional suppression increased the amount of mood disturbance our patients experienced. As it turned out, emotional control was positively related to emotional distress. Thus, those who were preoccupied with their disease and who kept tight control over their affective expression tended to be more, rather than less, anxious and depressed.

These findings indicate that efforts to control negative emotion do not work–those who tried hardest to suppress their depression were nonetheless more depressed. While we cannot make causal inferences from these data, since those who were more depressed may have been trying harder to suppress their feelings, the data suggest that efforts to keep control of the expression of emotions about cancer are counterproductive. Those who try to keep sadness, anxiety, anger, and other so-called negative emotions out of consciousness wind up more depressed and anxious despite, or in part because of, these efforts.

It might be thought that to the extent that such conscious or habitual efforts at shunning negative emotion work, such individuals might be, if anything, more happy than those who accept their negative feelings as they come. In fact, we found the opposite to be true among metastatic breast cancer patients. Those who avoided negative emotion suffered more of it. Indeed there is a danger that such patients may appear to be the best adjusted, because they try to show so little of their distress. Doctors may be misled into thinking they are doing fine, when in fact they are suffering in silence. In addition, they may receive less encouragement and support in living with their illness because friends and family are not fully aware of the extent of their distress. Indeed, one productive use of group interaction is to examine the mixed message such people convey.

Mary complained that her husband never seemed to take the time and effort to comfort her, either brushing her off or changing the topic. Yet the therapist had observed that she deflected any attention directed toward her problems, and continued to complain about her husband while failing to acknowledge the obvious efforts of several group members to comfort her. The therapist said, "Mary, you seem sad now but clearly do not want to talk about your sadness. Several group members have tried to reach out to you, but I wonder if they feel acknowledged for it." At this point several group members concurred, but provided excuses for Mary. The therapist went on: "I don't know how to help you. What could I do that would make you feel better?"

For the first time, Mary acknowledged that she appreciated the help that had been offered her, but did not like to take the time of the group to deal with her sadness. The intervention brought the problem of conflict over expressing emotion into the room—it became a group issue rather than one with her husband, and helped her to become more congruent in her overt and covert expression of emotion.

This is not to say that emotional restraint comes solely from patient ambivalence about identifying or expressing feelings. For a variety of reasons patients may feel genuine pressure to appear strong and able to cope with their situation. They often interpret this to mean that they should not show their real emotions and must maintain a positive attitude.

Partners and family members may unintentionally communicate the wish that the patient be strong because it helps them to avoid their own feelings of helplessness and fear. Other internal reasons for wanting to remain strong and in control may involve concerns about being overwhelmed with fear and anxiety.

The goal of supportive-expressive group therapy is for patients to be able to express all emotions, positive and negative. In this way they will not be hiding or denying any aspect of their experience. If negative affect is not allowed expression, a great deal of energy is required to suppress or bypass it. With its free expression, patients experience relief and encouragement as they find that they are also able to tolerate it. Finding that their emotions are tolerated by themselves and the group can give patients the courage to be more open and expressive with their loved ones.

FACILITATING EMOTIONAL
EXPRESSION IN THE GROUP

The experience of having faced the worst tends to make it less overwhelming, helping the patient to put it into some kind of new perspective. Even death itself, as we will discuss later, is less intimidating when confronted directly. Efforts to ward off awareness of threat are draining and counterproductive and impair the patient's ability to assess and manage the threat. On the other hand, supportive and open expression of fear, sadness, and other strong emotions tends to release their grip. Thus, by encouraging expression of disease-related emotion, therapists can facilitate better adjustment in their patients. We have found that support groups for cancer patients are an efficient and highly effective way to accomplish this.

"I'm good at this, this self-hypnosis, self-expression thing," said Susan. "So I sometimes just sit and feel how sad and scared I am. Sure it upsets me when someone dies in the group, but face it, we're all gonna die someday. Not because we're in the group, but because we have cancer. I'll take the sadness. Where can you go to just come unglued? You see, I'm crying now. Who knows why I'm crying?" Looking directly at the therapist, she quips, "Don't ask me why." "Moi?" responded the therapist, in mock surprise. "Who else can you come apart in front of and still feel okay about it? I can with my husband, he understands it, but it upsets him so much. I feel like melting him down. I'm not the woman he married—I've gained weight, I've got cancer, I'm not working." "You do so much for your family," responded several group members, "you raise your daughters, you're a beautiful wife." "I'm not the same," Susan continued. "I'm not the woman he married." After a pause, she added, "But I'm still a damned good cook." She and the group burst out laughing.

Laura was discussing the deterioration of her marriage—her husband had become openly involved with another woman. To add insult to injury, his family, which had been supportive of her, was becoming more alienated since her mother-in-law had died of cancer, implying to her that it was "odd" that she had survived cancer while their beloved mother had died. This was plenty to handle in the group, but the therapist noted a tear forming in Emily's eye. "What is it about Laura's story that is making you so sad?" he inquired. "My husband killed himself thirty years ago, and I still haven't gotten over my anger and disappointment in him. At the same time, I still miss being close with him."

Laura's recent loss of her husband had triggered reflections about Emily's long-standing one. They had found common ground, which helped Laura to better accept the group's suggestion that she had a right to be angry about her unceremonious exclusion from her husband's family in the wake of his abandonment of her. It was easier for her to become acquainted with this emotion through her identification with Emily than directly from her own experience—she was too "close" to it.

A crucial part of the leaders' work is to scan the group, looking for signs of emotion, and encourage that person to talk about it, vent the feelings, and share them with the group. Leaders should not always focus on the person who is talking, but rather scan the room for hints of sadness or anxiety—for example, a downturned gaze, a tear in the eye, some fidgeting. It is important that group leaders focus more on the affective than the cognitive flow of the group, the emotional environment more than the set of issues or problems addressed. This is, at first, a difficult skill to develop. Our training is such that we are taught to attend to the content of discussion, to follow the flow of logical thought, and complete one idea before moving on to the next. This is not so in running a support group. The goal is to encourage the development of a shared experience of common emotion: a pool of feelings in which the group immerses itself. Feelings are to be acknowledged, explored, identifed, openly discussed, and understood. As a mnemonic device, think of these steps in exploring emotions in groups in terms of the vowels in the alphabet: A-E-I-O-U.

1. Acknowledge affect.
2. Explore the emotion.
3. Identify the emotion.
4. Open expression to others.
5. Understand the emotion.

ACKNOWLEDGE AFFECT

Acknowledge the expression of emotion immediately. When group members take the lead and discuss their feelings, it is crucial that they sense that they have been heard and acknowledged. Every expression of feeling involves taking a risk, opening yourself up, and feeling vulnerable. Being rejected or ignored after such openness is a powerful message to keep feelings to themselves, not only to that person but to all group members. This undermines the therapeutic atmosphere of the group.

The husband of a cancer patient who had died two weeks earlier returned to the family group he had attended on a monthly basis to report about this final period of her life. He

had always been rather remote and logical, espousing the avoidance of difficult discus-
sions. Clearly, however, he needed to describe the ordeal he had been through. "It must
have been a terribly difficult time," said the therapist as a means of opening the door to
this discussion. "Not really," said Michael, overtly dismissing the therapist's observa-
tion but pursuing the opening anyway. "We never really discussed what was happen-
ing—I just spent a lot of time with her. The last week she was so weak that I just sat next
to her bed. I found myself reading nursery stories to her, as if she were a little child."

The sadness in the room was palpable, and the loneliness he felt was tem-
pered only by the fact that he was describing it to us. While he never overtly
agreed that sharing this sadness was a good idea, his heartfelt thanks at the
end of the session was indication enough.

Expressing and discussing a feeling, especially one related to cancer, involves risk taking. We identify our emotions more with our core being than
we do our thoughts. We are also strangely passive in relation to emotions—
they happen to us. As one support group member said: "We are responsible
for our thoughts, but not for our feelings." In discussing a feeling, a person
is reporting on an inner state, something he can choose to tell about or not,
but something he cannot choose not to have.

Yalom (1995) notes that the direct expression of feelings rather than
thoughts constrains defensive reactions: "The patient can devalue or ignore
them but cannot deny them, disagree with them, or take them away" (p.
166). He also adds that in difficult situations it can be extremely helpful for
the therapist to admit to having difficulties. He gives an example of running
a group of pediatric oncology nurses in which there was considerable tension between younger line nurses and older nurse managers. Although
warned that the situation was too hot to handle, he put it in terms of his own
dilemma in knowing whether or not to address this difficult issue. That led
to a fruitful discussion, because it involved an appropriate admission of the
therapist's discomfort as well as the content, which generated plenty of discomfort in the group as well. In this way, the therapist can model handling
internal conflict.

Richard was being vigorously treated for progressive and malignant pancreatic cancer.
He wanted to believe that the exceptionally aggressive treatment would put him "at the
end of the survival curve," but complained at the same time of being somewhat direc-
tionless. He had trouble initiating new projects, including planning special time with
his family despite their intense love for each other. Before his illness he had gone out of
his way to coach his daughter's softball team and drove his other daughter long dis-

tances to basketball tournaments. Why this inability to make full use of precious time? The therapist suspected that intensive planning meant to Richard that his days were really numbered, while living at random implied that he had plenty of time left. The therapist said, "Richard, I don't know quite what to do. I have the feeling that we need to discuss the possibility that this could be your last good summer with your family, and yet I don't know whether you want us to go there." Richard looked sad, but responded, "I think I need a kick in the pants. I hope there will be plenty more summers, but I guess if we make the most of this one and there are lots more, so much the better." He then went on to wonder aloud whether he should agree to his seventeen-year-old's request to spend the summer away from home. He had been inclined to send her away, acting as though they had all the time in the world. His ability to confront the possibility that his illness would progress rapidly allowed him to admit how much he wanted his older daughter near him.

When someone ventures a direct expression of feeling, it is important that it be directly acknowledged and reinforced. The lack of a response, or criticism, will be experienced as far more hurtful than the lack of comment after an observation or thought.

Richard felt somewhat uncomfortable in expressing his fear, but benefited from the experience in part because the therapist took a risk himself in exploring it, admitted to wondering if Richard could handle this exploration, and acknowledged how hard it was for Richard to face the worst possibilities.

The therapist admitting to feelings can be helpful, but other techniques also assist with the expression of emotion. It is often useful to simply restate the feeling the patient expressed so that the emotion is acknowledged and accepted.

"Jane, I am glad you told us how frightened you felt when you got the bad news about your bone scan. Can you tell us more about how you felt?"

Another approach is to elicit similar feelings from other group members who have been in similar situations:

"Perhaps others have had similar feelings after receiving some bad news. What was it like?"

These interventions acknowledge Jane's anxiety and allow her to pursue it further. They also facilitate the expression of similar feelings undoubtedly stirred up in others by her story. It is important that expression of others' experience complement rather than replace discussion of Jane's predicament. This is the difference between a kind of parallel play in which similar stories are presented in isolation or competition and a mutually reinforcing exploration of common emotion.

There are other useful ways for the therapist to acknowledge the expression of emotion, especially if other group members do not:

"I know it must have been hard for you to tell us how much this has been worrying you."
"I can hear how worried you are."
"Can you tell us what the worst part of it is for you?"

These interventions restate the emotion that has been expressed and invite the person to explore it further, providing both acknowledgment and encouragement.

EXPLORE EMOTION

A simple expression of feeling is a good start, but it is not enough to fully develop, understand, or resolve it. The next phase is to help the group members explore what the feeling is and then find a way to address it. The mere mention of a feeling does not do it justice—the patient expressing it must feel an emotional response to it, not merely a clarification or description.

In the cognitive-behavioral model, excessive emotion—depression, for example—is countered by cognition in the form of pointing out to the depressed patient that the selective focus on the negative only reinforces depression (Beck, 1995). However, when there is good reason for the patient's sadness or anxiety, a purely cognitive response by the group members or leaders can be experienced as dismissive, implying that the feeling is irrational. By contrast, an emotional response from another group member expressing a similar feeling validates the distress and helps the person work through it. Further, it conveys that she can be valued and cared about as a person not despite but because of her ability to express honestly what she is feeling. She does not have to put up a front, but rather elicits stronger support when she lets the barrier down. Indeed, such a patient can be made to feel that she is doing work for others in the group as well, as she helps them articulate and experience their own feelings.

Not all group members take to the discussion of feelings easily, and many may need some guidance in that direction. Consider the following example.

Several group members are discussing their fears about the cancer recurring and how each of them is struggling to cope with the anxiety that they may be facing a foreshortened future. One of the members who had been silent during the discussion interjects by saying, "I'm wondering if we can change the topic. I have a problem at work I'd like some help with." The therapist responds: "Before we do that, you haven't said anything throughout this discussion and I'm wondering how you've been feeling while we were talking about the fear of dying prematurely."

This is a good response because it does not allow the patient to change the topic before she has examined her emotional reaction to it.

You may be wondering at this point about whether a group member can ever change the topic of discussion without a challenge from the therapist. After all, members are taught to be assertive about using the group to get their needs met. Doesn't it make sense for anyone to have the right to change the direction of the discussion?

This is true, but this is also the reason that the therapist must be constantly scanning the group for its affective tone, more so than for the content of discussions. Clearly if there is a lull in the discussion, if there is no particular matter of emotional importance being discussed, it is quite reasonable for someone to bring up a new topic. The therapist needs to get the feel of the room, to sense when there is an emotional topic either on the floor or in the wings, and nurture its exploration. The sense of discomfort at leaving a feeling unresolved should be palpable to the therapist, and should guide the direction of the discussion.

The affect may seem overwhelming and may lead to group efforts to short-circuit it. It is the leaders' job to keep the affective flow intact.

Megan talked tearfully about what she had lost: "I was such a good therapist. I loved doing it, and I really felt I helped people. With the cancer now, I just can't do it anymore. That whole part of me is gone forever."

It might be tempting to try to cheer Megan up, with a "There, there, it's not so bad" kind of comment. This would only drive her sadness inward, making her feel that her loss isn't worth crying about, and certainly is not worth the time of the group. Instead, the group took her seriously.

"It is a real loss—your life is not the same," said the leader. Then Rebecca looked at Megan thoughtfully and said: "But you are our therapist. You are so articulate about

your feelings—you help me understand mine. And I get all this for free!" Rebecca chuckled. Laura added: "You express feelings for all of us. You still are helping people."

These comments were not false reassurance. They acknowledged Megan's loss, and her feelings about that loss, but in such a way that her loss was re-structured: Not everything was gone. She still used her therapeutic skill, but in a different way. In understanding and expressing her feelings, she was helping the other women in the group. Furthermore, they were responding to her vulnerability and sadness with warmth and caring—helping her in turn by acknowledging how much she helped them. The emotional flow was intact, even though discussions about lost careers and frustrated hopes were incomplete. The group response validated Megan's sadness and helped to put it into perspective. But a deeper issue was also addressed, one of Megan's sense of self-worth. Could she be of value if she was not functioning at her highest level? Could she be respected if she was not a professional? The emotional and social response conveyed to her that she was truly valued.

Megan smiled at Rebecca's comment about free treatment. "It's still not the same," she protested. "But, thank you for saying that—I'm glad if I can still do that for you."

Thus, the exploration of Megan's emotion leads to a deeper understanding of it, an acknowledgment of her willingness to share it with the group, and a response that helps her to put in into perspective.

IDENTIFY THE EMOTION

It often helps in dealing with an emotion to give it a name so that it becomes more understandable and less alien, as a variety of feelings may be mingled together, making it difficult to sort them out.

The group is engaged in a discussion of daily sources of stress and the women begin to talk about how this affects their health. One woman, Sue, begins to cry. The therapist asks her what the tears are about and she replies, "I'm so afraid of what this cancer is do-ing to me. I just can't handle it. I'm ... so ... frightened." She begins to sob uncontrol-lably. At this point, Sue has named the feeling, and the therapist reaffirms this and encourages her to pursue it further in more detail: "I know this can be difficult to look at, Sue, but it might be really helpful to you if you try to tell us more about some of the frightening thoughts you are having." Sue then said: "I don't know ... I—I'm afraid of the pain, of being alone, of leaving my children, of everything." At this point Sue is over-whelmed, and the therapist tries to help her examine each aspect of the feeling: "Let's try to look at these one at a time. Can you tell us more about your fear of the pain?"

The leader was determined to pursue Sue's anxiety and explore the compo-nents of it, which had the effect of making the reasons for her fear clearer as specific instances of her feelings emerged and were described. Furthermore, it made Sue feel cared about because of her fear, not despite it. Such exploration made the fear more immediate but at the same time more understandable. Furthermore, the other members of the group, in participating, can obviously identify with her, yet feel her fear in an attenuated form, mingled with con-cern for her, which gives them a greater sense of mastery over it. Thus the leader's job is to identify and clarify the feeling. It is often helpful to have the patient describe the situation that elicited it, especially if something in the group discussion triggered the response. This brings the feeling more into the "here-and-now," making it understandable for everyone.

In taking this approach the patient eventually was able to differentiate her fears about dying into pieces with which she could cope. She identified the aspects over which she had some control, such as dealing with pain and preparing her children in case the cancer progressed. She also began to ex-plore her related feelings of aloneness, and doing so in the group context helped to diminish them. Furthermore, an outpouring of concern from the therapist and group members helped to counter her sense of isolation in a concrete and immediate way.

It often happens in these groups that when members talk about feeling an-gry, they look and act sad. This incongruence between the experience and expression of emotion may lead to confusing responses from others. A hus-band may not understand how angry his wife is at him because each time she brings it up she cries. Or, as in the situation described below, the appar-ent absence of distress in a situation where there should be plenty can have the effect of deflecting support.

Laura is talking further about her husband, who had left her after fifteen years of mar-riage for another woman who works in the same office: "My husband says that he has 'done the cancer thing' with me, put up with all the worry and inconvenience and treat-ments and now he wants to enjoy himself. I still love him. In fact, I love him more now than I ever did before. I'm sure I'll get him back—there's already trouble in paradise [his new relationship]."

The events are stark, and clearly there must be feelings about them. But they are missing. Where is the anger and hurt and fear about the future? The therapist has a choice at this point—to pursue and try to deepen the expression of emotion regarding this feeling, or to turn to the group for their empathic emotional response. In this case, the therapist feels that Laura is too closed to (and close to) the obvious emotions elicited by her situation, so she turns to others in the group.

> The therapist says, "I wonder how others feel listening to Laura's story." Kelly (with tears rolling down her cheeks) responds: "I just can't believe it. I thought of you as the model couple. When my husband was talking about writing a book about being the husband of a breast cancer patient, the first person I told him to talk to was Ralph [Laura's husband]. It scares me about being alone as I get sicker. If Ralph could do this to you, I can only imagine what my husband would do, given how he talks. We'll be going down the street and he'll say: 'Would that be a good one for me to marry after you're gone?'"

Here Kelly is doing some affective work of her own, but for Laura as well, feeling both for herself and for Laura the hurt that comes with a sense of betrayal. She names the fear of being left alone by a husband she had thought she could count on, even though at this point Laura cannot do it.

> Then Jill added: "It makes me so mad. Didn't he ever hear of wedding vows—until death do us part? He acts like he's been doing you a favor. You've been doing him a favor. You're better off without the SOB."
>
> Laura continued to deny the hurt and anger lurking below the surface of her story, but directed some of it at the "other woman." However, she heard from the group that anger, fear, and sadness were names to be applied to what must be feelings.

During the next month, she became more overtly sad and angry as she kept the group apprised of what was happening. There was less tension in the group's perception of a gap between what she said and what she felt. In naming these feelings and bringing them together with the events of her life, she also opened herself up more to allowing the group to comfort and help her. Whereas at first she took the stance that she had it all figured out and knew she would get him back, over the weeks she came to more openly accept this great loss and the group's help with it. The process of naming the feelings associated with her situation had the effect of clarifying the reasons for their existence and her right to have them. Her initial denial that she was hurt or angry constituted an attempt to minimize her recognition of the damage that had been done to her. As she identified her hurt and anger, she was better able to accept and respond to her new situation, and she received more help from the group in doing so.

OPEN THE EMOTIONAL FIELD TO OTHERS

Encourage mutual and multiple expressions of emotion. It is also important to facilitate the discussion of feelings elicited in other group members in response to the initial show of feelings. When one person in a room expresses emotion, it is (and should be) difficult for others not to respond emotionally, perhaps with similar feelings, perhaps with contrary ones.

Groups work best when leaders make the expression of emotion a common, fluid, and shared experience, rather than a structured, individual, or sequential one. Group therapy is not simply a series of individual therapeutic interventions with witnesses. Rather it is an interactive process in which the interplay is far more than the sum of the individual parts. Indeed, one of the great opportunities in group therapy is the development of emotional resonance,* a situation in which one person's emotion triggers the expression of related feelings in others.

> Megan started out discussing a recent fight with her husband Dave, whom she felt had not been attentive enough to her progressing illness. Megan began to cry and said, "I always have this fear that I will be left alone, that no one will really want to look after me when I get sick. I know that Dave has been pretty good about it, but I can't stand it when I sense him pulling back."
>
> The therapist saw this as an opportunity to explore the group's feelings about Megan, rather than speculate about Dave's reaction to her. He asked, "How are others in the group feeling about Megan right now?"
>
> Rebecca said, "We are not going to let you drift away from us. You give so much to us. I can't conceive of leaving you alone as you get sicker. Where could you go to talk about how you feel with so many people, and not have them tell you, 'Just get on with it.' That is what we are here for."
>
> The therapist then checked in with Megan, asking if she felt Rebecca's concern for her. Megan responded, "Yes, I know it is there, and it makes me feel good. I know some of my fear is irrational, but it is always there."

---

*We are indebted to Dr. Anne Harrington of Harvard University for this term.

By eliciting comments from the group members, Megan felt supported and that her feelings were accepted yet challenged. She was also given some helpful ideas on how she might talk to her husband about the issue.

As we discussed in Chapter 4, emotional expression is facilitated by the use of here-and-now techniques in the group. Feelings expressed about people outside the room, even important people in a person's life, are less intense than those involving interactions in the room. As Yalom (1995) puts it: "The process focus is the power cell of the group!" (p. 137).

> A group of metastatic breast cancer patients were in an unusually feisty mood. Considerable bickering emerged, including squabbles between members who usually got along quite well. The therapist noted the unusual emotional climate, and wondered aloud whether the feelings might have to do with the recent death of a member who had only come to the group a few times. Perhaps the group was feeling a double loss— Miriam's death and the sense that she had slipped away before they had a chance to get to know her. The tone in the room changed, and the group got down to the unfinished business of grieving a dimly perceived loss.

This intervention required identifying the affect in the group, naming it, and raising a question about its source. The therapist hypothesized that the anger was both a recognition and an avoidance of grief. Often group process can be used to illuminate problems with other relationships outside of the group. The key is to stimulate discussion of feelings in the room and to use the outside problem as a template. Keep the focus in the room.

> Irene complained bitterly that her husband simply did not understand her: "I tell him how hard it is for me to go to chemotherapy every other day and then come home, feel terrible, and try to do the housework. He just looks bored." My problems are all mine— he acts as though I should be able to handle it. I don't know why I even bother talking to him. What good does it do?"
>
> The therapist acknowledged the feeling, but brought the discussion into the room: "Irene, are you feeling helped in here?"

This question changes the direction of the discussion. Some of the problem may indeed be the husband's lack of interest or response, but he is not there. Some of it may be that the patient is inconsolable, or feels that no one cares about her.

"I don't know what good it does to talk. Who wants to listen to me anyway? I'm just a burden."

The focus is now moving into the room, and multiple involved people are available.

"We want to help," says Julie. "I feel the same way sometimes. I'm just too tired to do anything, but I feel so useless when I can't even help the kids with schoolwork and cook dinner. I understand your frustration."

This is an empathic response, but Irene just looks frustrated, and does not acknowledge Julie's response.

The therapist pursues the response further:

"How did you feel after Julie talked?"

This can help Irene notice that she does not feel helped even when assistance is offered, and the whole group can see it.

"I don't know. I guess it made me feel a little better."

The therapist continued: "Julie, did you know that your words had helped Irene?"

"I wasn't sure," she responded. "I had hoped they would, but I wasn't sure you heard me."

This kind of exchange helps Irene to see that she may be discouraging her husband from responding to her because he gets so little acknowledgment of his efforts. It would be mere speculation to say this in the abstract, but bringing the feelings into the room makes it clearer, and mobilizes the feelings of more than one group member.

"Thanks, Julie. It feels good to be understood."

The principle of sharing feelings around the room should not be used to short-circuit a given patient's expression and exploration of her own feelings. This is a delicate balance, and therapists need to develop a sense for when a second expression of emotion amplifies rather than replaces the initial patient's feeling. A key guideline is whether the discussion as a whole is continuing or dampening the exploration of feeling, and whether the patient who started the process is feeling acknowledged or avoided. Sometimes it is tempting to reinforce the commonality of experience among group members, thereby normalizing a given person's reaction. Done too soon, however, this shortcuts the expression of feeling and creates a kind of artificial agreement that may not reflect the experience of group members. Pain must be borne and expressed before it can be shared and understood.

> Sue had two more cycles to go in a very vigorous course of chemotherapy. She had suffered various side effects from the treatments, and stated that she was "exhausted" and felt she "just can't take any more treatment."

One possible response often relied upon in support groups is the camaraderie of common experience. Others could say at this point, "Oh, yes, I felt exhausted too," and the discussion could drift toward the rigors of chemotherapy and its side effects. Instead the therapist decides to pursue Sue's response further:

> "The treatment has been very hard on you, and it seems as if you're feeling especially bad right now. When you are feeling this bad, it is hard to believe you will ever get out of it. Do you remember ever feeling this way before? How did you deal with it then?"

This response helped Sue to recall previous times when her treatment got her down and how she eventually was able to pull herself out of her despair. It reminded her that the present is not a necessary predictor of the future—the course of her illness may be up and down rather than steadily downhill. It also enabled her to assure herself that her feelings of exhaustion were temporary.

UNDERSTAND THE EMOTION

> " . . . mere catharsis is not in itself a corrective experience. Cognitive learning or restructuring (much of which is provided by the therapist) seems necessary for the patient to be able to generalize group experiences to outside life. . . . Without the acquisition of some knowledge about the general patterns in interpersonal relationships, the patient may, in effect, have to rediscover the wheel in each subsequent interpersonal interaction." (Yalom, 1995, p. 216)

The expression of emotion is a means but not an end in itself in supportive-expressive group therapy. Such experiences are at times painful, often taxing, and to be worth the effort they must be a source of learning. As Sullivan said: "The magic occurs in the interpersonal relations, and the real magic is done by the patient, not by the therapist. The therapist's skill and art lie in keeping things simple enough so that something can happen; in other words, he clears the field for favorable change, and then tries to avoid getting in the way of its development" (Sullivan, 1954, p. 227). Many situations stimulate affect; groups provide an opportunity for observation as well as participation.

Exploring emotion can be an important means of clarifying problems, depriving them of some of their hold on the person by illuminating their source. Anxiety is worse than fear, depression more debilitating than sadness. The process of uncovering emotion can refine and clarify it.

> *Martha recounted a rather harrowing story of her husband having told her that she was "looking fat" and that she should "go sleep on the couch." The remarkable thing was that she did. She said, "Well, I've lost six pounds. I've been very careful about my weight, but I guess I am bloating in the evening." Only later did she begin to realize how inappropriate and nasty her husband had been, and she eventually returned to her bedroom (but only after he finally unlocked the door). However, it still was difficult for her to realize how insulting this was.*

As we discussed this episode, Martha realized that the therapist did not think she had done the right thing by retreating to the living room rather than getting in touch with her understandable anger at her husband. Another patient in the group wondered aloud whether Martha was feeling criticized by the therapist. She acknowledged that she was. We then observed that she was responding in the group the way she had with her husband, absorbing our response to her situation with guilt as justifiable criticism, rather than sharing our anger at her husband ("What's wrong with me?" rather than "What's wrong with him?"). The therapist went on to discuss a recent family group meeting in which her husband had made a rather hostile comment about the therapist's appearance. "Yes, that's the word," said Martha. "Hostile." Her focus on guilt rather than anger had deflected her recognition of how devaluing her husband had been, and the interaction with the group helped to clarify it and propelled her toward more assertiveness with him.

At other times, anger is not the hidden emotion, but actually the cover for anxiety and fear.

Irene was the image of what every cancer patient fears. She had become painfully thin, could only walk with assistance, and because of metastases to her brain, was losing motor control and was unable to hold her head upright. She sat in the group with her head wobbling, until one of the therapists held it for her. She talked with the group about her worsening condition, and her plans for her death. Because she felt so weak, she left the group early.

Considerable anger emerged after she left: "How could she come in that condition?" "Why does she push herself so hard?"

Here the therapist's intervention was crucial: "What are we so angry about?" he wondered aloud. The emotion reverberating around the room was named and its meaning was questioned.

The members seemed to be angry at her. But as the discussion proceeded, it became clear that they were really angry at the illness they shared and their fear of it. Once one predominant emotion had been named, others were free to surface.

One member then said: "I admire her. I hope that when I am that ill I will have the courage to go where I want to go."

Thus tolerating the expression of anger allowed another emotion to emerge, and it helped to put the anger in perspective. She represented one thing that frightened them, but something else that inspired them.

Indeed they made a plan to meet in her home the following week, which they did, shortly before she died.

THERAPISTS' EMOTIONS
AND TRANSPARENCY

Openness and emotional expressiveness are a central goal of this treatment. Facilitating them may be the hardest thing for therapists to learn. Tolerating someone else's sadness, anxiety, fear, or anger is not easy. They tend to arouse comparable or complementary emotions in the therapist, and the tendency is to want to act quickly to reestablish emotional equilibrium—your own (a countertransference reaction) and that of the patient.

Medical training is often an endless exercise in affect suppression. It is considered unprofessional to have an emotional reaction to a situation that would clearly induce feeling. Should a doctor or nurse cry at the death of a patient (why not?). A reaction of disgust or fear could very well hamper effective work in the emergency department or operating room; but we in medicine tend to overdo it. Here is the way a daughter's natural reaction to her father's untimely death was handled at one city hospital during my (D.S.) training.

> *A fourteen-year-old girl dissolved in tears and began screaming, "No, no, it can't be true. He's not dead," when she saw doctors discontinue their resuscitation efforts on her father, who had just died of liver failure. Rather than taking her into a more private setting and allowing her to continue her grief, someone called for a shot of Valium for the girl. I objected, saying that she was doing what she needed to do, and that if she didn't she would be looking for psychiatric help later. Since I was just a medical student at the time, my opinion was brusquely overruled: "She is upsetting the other patients." "If this bothers you, you take the Valium," I added, not so diplomatically.*

It seems as if we treat crying in medicine as if it were bleeding. We are trained to treat a hemorrhage by applying direct pressure until it stops. The therapist must learn the discipline of accepting and encouraging emotion rather than following the natural tendency to prematurely reassure, avoid, or distract from its expression. When a patient is upset, don't just do something, stand there.

Emotions in patients tend to trigger emotions in therapists. At times they are similar; at other times, surprisingly complementary. In Table 6.1 we show some common examples.

These are meant to be suggestive rather than definitive. The main point is that an empathic response in the therapist is not necessarily identical to the patient's emotion. Depressed patients frequently make others angry, for example. You want to shake them by the shoulders and say: "Things are not really as bad as that. Get on with it." If, as a therapist, you find yourself frequently angry with a patient, ask yourself whether the patient may be depressed. Being able to identify such feelings may help you to manage and control your own immediate responses. They will seem less alien and trou-

TABLE 6.1   Examples of Patients' Emotions Triggering Therapists' Emotions

Patient's Emotion	Therapist's Emotion
Sadness	Sadness
Depression	Anger
Fear	Fear
Anxiety	Anxiety
Anger	Fear
Happiness	Happiness
Sexual arousal	Anxiety

bling, and allow you to further pursue the patient's affect with less concern about containing your own.

What about the therapists' feelings? How are they to be dealt with? Should therapists always emote? Does that help or hinder the therapeutic process? For example, is it destructive for a therapist to cry when talking about the death of a group member?

> "Ask yourself, 'Where is the group now? Is it a concealed, overly cautious group that may profit from a leader who models personal self-disclosure? Or has it already established vigorous self-disclosure norms and is in need of other assistance?' First of all consider whether your behavior will interfere with your group-maintenance function. You must know when to recede into the backgound. Unlike the individual therapist, the group therapist does not have to be the fulcrum of therapy. In part, the therapist is midwife to the group: you must set a therapeutic process in motion and take care not to interfere with that process by insisting on your centrality." (Yalom, 1995, p. 216)

The expression of emotion, the revelation of inner feelings by therapists, is not an end itself; rather it should be a means to an end. If the expression of emotion helps patients in need of such assistance to open up and examine their own feelings, it can be useful. If it directs attention away from the patients' problems toward the therapists', it is a bad idea.

If the group is grieving the loss of a member, and the therapist is moved to tears by discussing it, so be it. As long as the therapist's open sadness continues rather than disrupts the flow of emotion in the room, it can be viewed as a sign of compassion and involvement. However, it must not distract from the ongoing work of the group or imply that the therapist is not able or willing to continue his or her leadership role.

As a therapist you are asking patients in the group to do some of the most difficult things in life. In the midst of dealing with a life-threatening illness, you are asking them to discuss the hurt, fear, and pain, look their fears right in the eye, with the promise that they will ultimately feel better, more prepared, more active in the face of their illnesses. Is it not reasonable that these patients ask something difficult of you, challenge you to do something hard as well? They will ask if you know what you are are doing, if you feel uncomfortable about the path you are charting for them. They will test your concern for them—do you really care about them?

The challenge may come in the form of noting differences:

"How can you understand what it is like for us to have breast cancer—you're not a woman and you don't have cancer."

In this situation the therapist is being pushed away and his role is being challenged. The skill is in acknowledging the challenge and responding to it without being pushed even farther away, or trying to immediately build a bridge over the distance rather than repair the break in the road:

Therapist: "It is true I don't have breast cancer (although men can actually get it). And I am sure I have a lot more to learn about what it means to have it—I hope you'll teach me. But one of the things I've learned already is that none of us knows for sure who will be around next week. The real issue is not whether I am going through the same thing— clearly I am not—but rather whether I can understand enough to be of help. What else do I need to know?"

Not uncommonly, some group therapists actually do have the same illness as the members. This provides a natural bond, but it is important that the therapist not assume that she or he knows just what the members are going through. Therapists' intuition is likely to be good, but it may not be. Also, they are in a dual role, and must remember that there may be group process reasons for the group seeing the therapists as removed that need exploration, regardless of their personal base of experience with the illness. Avoid making assumptions about commonality or difference, but do explore.

Indeed, it is possible to have *pseudoempathy,* to presume a connection that is not there. It is dangerous to assume that because the therapist is in a similar situation, he or she really knows the patient's current dilemma. Pseudoempathy can also preclude further discussion and deny the validity of the group members' sense of separateness. In addition, the therapist's discussion of personal medical or other problems must not undermine the group's ability to express anger, disappointment, or other emotions regarding the therapist's performance. Self-disclosure on the part of the therapist must not turn into a plea for sympathy or a retreat from the reasonable expectations of the group.

There will, however, be times when further self-disclosure is helpful. The key is whether the therapist's self-disclosure involves his or her work in the group, or something else. Disclosure within the domain of the group can be very helpful; outside of such boundaries it can be a distraction.

Sometimes there are situations that occur in the therapist's immediate life that cannot be ignored by the group because of its thematic similarity:

A close friend of the therapist's had been dying of a brain tumor over the preceding two years of the group. The therapist came to a group meeting directly from his friend's funeral. His sadness was obvious, and the group inquired solicitously about his feelings. "I have lost someone who was like a brother to me. It makes me feel helpless and sad. I did everything I could to help him and his family, but the sense that nothing further is possible, no more conversations, no more jokes, no more tears, is very much with me today." The group responded with considerable concern. For a few minutes, the tables were turned and they ministered to the therapist. The group's healing balm—concern for the feelings of one of them—was generously applied. After about twenty minutes, the issue had been discussed, and the therapist began to inquire about how various members of the group were doing, and they got on to their concerns.

Such instances occur, and the willingness of therapists to be appropriately open can move the group forward. At the same time, the focus should never stay for long on the problems or situation of the therapist, other than in his or her role as therapist. As Harry Stack Sullivan observed (Sullivan, 1954), both psychotherapist and patient have problems, but psychotherapy is a process whereby they focus on the problems of the patient.

As Yalom notes (1995), the right kind of emotional disclosure is welcomed by patients, and the wrong kind is not desired:

"I have often posed this question [what further information should therapists have provided?] to patients at the end of therapy. The great majority express the wish that the therapist had been more open, more personally engaged in the group. Very few would

have wanted therapists to have discussed more of their private life or personal problems with them. The therapist, I think, need not fear being stripped and asked to stand shivering and naked before the group. Furthermore, there is evidence that leaders are more transparent than they know." (Yalom, 1995, p. 211)

Patients often sense more about the therapist's emotional response than the therapist thinks is visible, and they appreciate open acknowledgment of those feelings. They don't necessarily want to know more about the therapist's life outside of the group, but they are keenly interested in his or her life inside the group.

One obvious corollary of the importance of patients sharing emotion openly is that co-therapists need to do the same thing. Occasionally this will happen during the group, especially if there is an important disagreement, misunderstanding, or bruised feelings. Typical sources of discomfort are one therapist stepping on the other's interventions by making a comment or interpretation immediately after the other therapist has said something. This has the effect of canceling out or negating what the other therapist has just said, and can lead to some tension. Often, on the other hand, co-therapists will tune in to rather different aspects of group function, discussion, and emotion, which can prove quite helpful.

We strongly recommend a half hour of debriefing after a ninety-minute group to allow co-therapists to review what happened, discuss any emotional issues between them, assess how individual patients are doing, and make plans for the future. Such discussions are helped by the willingness of co-therapists to be nondefensive and direct with each other, for example, "When you said that Mary seemed sad rather than angry, I felt brushed aside, since I had just made an observation about her anger." Such discussions can help co-therapists work out stronger collaborative relationships, and avoid working at cross-purposes in the group.

CONCLUSION

Mobilizing the expression of emotion is a crucial part of the therapists' work. They must constantly scan the room, look for signs of feelings, elicit and acknowledge them, and use them constructively to help members become more involved with each other and to learn from their feelings. Thus there is a progression from acknowledging to exploring, identifying, searching for similar or reactive feelings in others, and understanding such emotions. Feelings are not right or wrong, they simply are. They may be rational or irrational, but they can be better understood and dealt with when they are expressed rather than suppressed, and they are a crucial focus of supportive-expressive group therapy.

PART THREE
HELPING PATIENTS
MANAGE THEIR
EXISTENTIAL CONCERNS

CHAPTER 7

Dealing with Dying

The best antidote to the fear of nonbeing is being with.

THE EXISTENTIAL ORIENTATION

There is a deep irony to the temporal focus of psychotherapies with an existential orientation, especially those that help people deal with life-threatening illnesses. Traditional psychoanalytically oriented psychotherapies focus primarily on the past—on how a person's upbringing influences character development and how parental introjects color current interpersonal relationships. Understanding the past, through corrective experiences in the transference with the therapist, is meant to improve the present and the future.

The existential orientation is to the future rather than the past, focusing on the contingency of life and its fragility. Yalom (1980, 1995) describes these ultimate concerns of existence: "death, isolation, freedom, and meaninglessness" (1995, p. 91). As the future becomes shorter, the therapeutic emphasis on it becomes greater. To focus on the past would be a retreat from the threat of death, a pretense that childhood could be relived and life redesigned. Rather, the imminent threat of death becomes the main focus in such psychotherapies. The less future there is, the more important it becomes.

The term *existential* in philosophy refers to the point of view which holds that there is no *essence* of human consciousness separate from existence. The vulnerable, transitory nature of existence is not a bug in the program—rather this fragility is inherent in the beauty and meaning of life. The more people face this fragility, the more they live authentically. Thus, dealing with death is not only a necessity, it is an opportunity to sort out the important things in life. Furthermore, doing so in support groups can in the process enhance the other three ultimate concerns:

1. Isolation, through enhanced caring and connection with other members of the group;
2. Freedom, through recognizing that important choices are still to be made about how members live the remainder of their lives;
3. Meaning, through using their lives as an example to help other group members, family, and friends cope with their own mortality.

The concerns of isolation, freedom and meaning are discussed in Chapter 8.

The therapeutic task is to facilitate members' open discussion of death and dying. To the extent that death can be "detoxified," it is to be done by facing rather than avoiding it. For most cancer patients, death raises a number of separate concerns that are experienced emotionally as one overwhelming and unmanageable problem. In addition to facilitating the expression of emotions and providing emotional support, the therapist helps patients break down this difficult topic into a series of separate and more manageable issues (Spiegel and Glafkides, 1983; Spiegel and Yalom, 1978).

DISCUSSING DYING

As mentioned in the Introduction, one of us (D.S.) had occasion to present this line of research to the Dalai Lama when he visited Stanford University. I asked him why he felt that facing death so directly seemed to be more comforting than frightening. He smiled in his childlike but profound way and responded: "I have a very busy travel schedule." I feared at this point that we were not communicating, despite his excellent command of English. He continued: "It makes me anxious, and when I feel particularly nervous I call one of my assistants and ask him what I will be doing for the next three days. He tells me and I feel better. That is the way we Buddhists feel about death. We make it familiar territory to us, and it becomes less frightening."

In the same way, making the discussion of death everyday fare deprives it of some of its shock value. It is the job of the therapists to bring hidden fears into the light of day, to make them visible and able to be discussed. Thus, when a patient makes a comment about adverse results from a diagnostic test, the therapist should pursue the line of thinking that undoubtedly follows the bad news: "This must have made you worried that the cancer is progressing more rapidly than you had hoped?" Such a question gives the patient an opportunity to express fears about early mortality. Another way to develop the discussion is to say something like: "So death must feel closer now." This conveys to the group that you are willing to discuss their deepest fears. It is important that the therapist not get too far ahead, implying that he or she knows something the patient does not know about the implications of the tests. Nonetheless, it is important to lead in the direction of exploring the inherent meaning of bad news.

Death is one of the major themes of support groups for patients with life-threatening illness. Whenever it comes up, it is worthy of discussion. When the condition of a group member deteriorates, it is important for the group leaders to comment on that fact and to invite discussion. When a group member is missing from a meeting, it is crucial to note the absence and to inquire about the health of the missing person. This reassures those present that they, too, will not slip away unnoticed. When a group member dies, grieving that person is the work of the group. The therapist's role is to be sure that the elephant in the room—the yet-unnamed fear evoked because a member is missing, someone has gotten bad news about a test, or someone has recently died—is discussed rather than ignored. Yalom describes this core existential conflict as "the tension between the awareness of the inevitability of death and the wish to continue to be" (1980, p. 8). The concern about dying from the disease is usually the most difficult issue for cancer patients to address.

One of the leading objections to the formation of support groups for people with life-threatening illnesses is the concern that they will be frightened and demoralized by the deterioration and death of other members of the group. Such losses are inevitable and painful and if they are not handled well the effect could well be demoralizing. Nonetheless, the danger of such problems is greatly exaggerated, especially in comparison with the opportunity such losses afford for useful exploration of unavoidable fears about dying and death. The fundamental premise of supportive-expressive group therapy is that all serious problems related to illness are better dealt with openly and directly, and death is the ultimate example of this.

Fearful as death is, familiarity takes away some of its sting. Therapists can be especially helpful in picking up hints of death anxiety and making them overt. Any mention of death deserves further exploration, even at the expense of other important material in the group. Therapists can help by inquiring about the effect of previous losses: "It has been a month since Mary died. I wonder how people are feeling about it now."

Isolation amplifies death anxiety, so encourage group discussion about death. Strangely, the best response to the threat of nonbeing is being with, since so much of the core comprehension of death comes in the form of isolation (Yalom, 1980; Spiegel, 1993b). The therapist aims to make it easier for members to voice their anxieties and fears, with the full acknowledgment of one's essential aloneness in facing mortality. Yet the process of the group discussion is meant to counter the experience of isolation stimulated by the content of the discussion. It is critically important to feel cared about at moments when one contemplates the ultimate isolation, death itself.

Indeed, frank discussion of death anxiety provokes a kind of paradox: The very thought of being completely alone, of dying, is a common bond; group members are together in facing the threat of isolation. As one member discusses her dread of dying, she is comforted by the concern of others, and also by the similarity of their anxieties. One of the ways in which we comprehend the concept of death in a personal sense is through separation from loved ones (Yalom, 1980). Many of our cultural metaphors for death involve being alone. Social processes that isolate those threatened with death only intensify death anxiety. Being alone with fears of death makes you feel dead already, removed from those who provide care and comfort. This can be experienced as a foretaste of the future, a chilling sense of absolute aloneness. Those with cancer are extremely sensitive to the withdrawal of support from family, friends, and physicians.

Conversely, intense and personal discussion, especially about death itself, creates a strong bond that makes patients feel less alone with their fears, and more alive. The process of discussing fears of death, which can be quite intense, mitigates rather than reinforces dread about dying and death, whereas the process of avoidance and denial of the topic tends to reinforce feelings of isolation as though one were already dead.

"What can you as therapist do in the face of the inevitable? I think the answer lies in the verb to be. You do by being, by being there with the patient. Presence is the hidden agent of help in all forms of therapy. Patients looking back on their therapy rarely remember a single interpretation you made, but they always remember your presence, that you were there with them. The group configuration is not you, the therapist, and they, the dying;

it is we who are dying, we who are banding together in the face of our common condition. The group well demonstrates the double meaning of the word apartness: we are separate, lonely, apart from but also a part of. One of my members put it elegantly when she described herself as a lonely ship in the dark. Even though no physical mooring could be made, it was nonetheless enormously comforting to see the light of other ships sailing the same water." (Yalom, 1995 p. 96)

EXPOSURE TO COPING
WITH DYING

Avoidance of death deprives cancer patients of an opportunity to see how well others can cope with the fear of death. Even the ultimate threat of non-being can be faced with considerable fortitude, and it encourages patients to see others who can look death right in the eye, manage their dread, and live life well.

One physician with breast cancer said in a support group, "There is something reassuring about knowing the exact manner of your death. I no longer have all those questions about how it will happen. I know. It is like a 95-year-old woman in the village where I grew up. She knew she would die soon, and was completely unafraid."

In another support group Marie, an artist, described her recent experience watching a friend die of cancer: "It wasn't ugly. For the first time I could see that I could do it. I knew after watching her that I could do it too. It wasn't wonderful but it wasn't that terrible."

Being a witness and having the privilege of helping someone through the dying process is a special gift to both the dying patient and those who cared for her.

Pam, a slender, attractive, executive secretary, was endlessly helpful and supportive to others. She took on the task of updating the group membership list. She asked how others were doing, visited the dying, called people to check on them, and was genuinely caring. For reasons that never became clear, because she was such a pleasant, attractive person, she had not married, but had a circle of friends and a caring family. However, she always put herself last. Her brother had been dying for some time, and at the end of one meeting Pam said, almost casually, "It's been a rough time for me ever since my brother died three weeks ago." The group was flabbergasted that she had not mentioned it sooner, and perhaps a bit guilty as well that no one had asked her.

As Pam lay dying in the hospital, the group rallied for her. The therapist arrived at the hospital hours before she died. Her sister made a point of telling the therapist how a visit from two group members several days before had resulted in a transformation of Pam. She had been admitted the previous week, and had been quite anxious. She had been having trouble breathing, and was panicked at the thought of dying, despite having carefully written a will and having talked about her impending death with everyone close to her. She even discussed it with the children to whom she volunteered time. Several had come to see her in the hospital. However, she had not been able to bring herself to make her funeral arrangements. There was something about the concreteness of this final act that had been just too much for her. Megan and Rebecca arrived Saturday evening and had a talk with her. "How much time do I have?" she asked. "I'm no good at lying, and I don't know for sure," replied Megan. "Maybe days, maybe weeks. There is one more thing you have to do. You have to let us know what your wishes are in regard to handling your body—it will help your family." Pam chose cremation. Her sister said to the therapist: "After that, she became calm. That discussion did something for her. And the group members were here all the time—they were so helpful." Thus, finally Pam received some of what she had given.

Often members become quite close during the final stages of life. We have found it useful to offer to have a group meeting in the home of a dying member. The group is reaching out, and it enables them to remain in contact after the dying person can no longer make it to the group. Clearly the member and her family must agree and participate in making the arrangements.

The breast cancer support group met in Rebecca's home twice before she died. The comfort and care shown by her family (mother, husband, and daughters) were obvious. Rebecca talked about her older daughter's plans to take a job in the Bay Area rather than the East Coast to be near her. Rebecca was trying to be neutral about it: "Well, okay if she really wants to and it is good for her career." The group chided her gently: "Don't you really want her nearby?" they asked. "Yes," she replied. "Then don't worry about it. She is a grown woman, now. She can tell you no if she needs to—be sure you let her know what you want."

At the second meeting, this time in her bedroom rather than the living room, she sat holding the hand of a new member in the group, making sure she was comfortable and felt accepted. This was just days before her death. The model of her openness to others, making the group feel welcomed, encouraged everyone else. After she had died, many members commented on how poised and caring for others she was right until the end. "I hope I can be like that," a number of people commented.

Seeing group members and others through the process of dying has a number of consequences. Obviously, those with life-threatening illnesses attend to others with the thought "There but for the grace of God go I." Some will have had experiences of loved ones dying of cancer, and may be imprinted with the belief that their dying will be just as horrible as that of their mother, sister, or uncle. Strangely enough, however, the more deaths they see, the more they come to understand that there is no "one" way to die with cancer, that there are multiple possible pathways of dying, some more peaceful than others, some more painful than others, some slower than others. The very range of exposure allows group members to start wondering about what constitutes a "good" death. Indeed, most cancer patients fear the process of dying more than death itself (Spiegel and Yalom, 1978; Spiegel and Glafkides, 1983; Spiegel, 1993b). The criteria that often emerge for a "good" death fall in two categories:

FAMILY
    A. having the opportunity to set things straight with important people
    B. saying "good-bye"
    C. being comfortable in one's home
    D. being surrounded by loved ones
    E. not feeling a burden to the family

MEDICAL
    A. freedom from pain
    B. having control over treatment decisions
    C. avoiding heroic treatment measures

When these and other aspects of dying are discussed openly, they transform death from an overwhelming threat to a challenge—something to be faced and handled rather than avoided.

One woman returned to her group after the sudden death of her cousin, also of cancer. She reported to the group: "I spent a lot of time with her. I'm glad I did—I was able to help out—more than others because I knew what she was going through. The strange thing is that I feel calmer about death now than I did before I saw her die. Why? I watched her go through it, and I thought to myself, "I can do this. I can get through something like this. It isn't wonderful, but I can see that I can handle it."

After a while, many groups come to be on intimate terms with death and with one another in the face of it. They often use humor to express this familiarity:

Pam and her brother used to talk openly about their illnesses (her breast cancer and his heart disease) and their similarly poor prognoses: "At the end of the last phone call, my brother told me we were in a 'dead heat.'" We all laughed. Pam died several months after her brother.

Group members can learn to discover in one another an ability to handle even the most difficult issue in life with clarity and dignity, and feel stronger for it.

"What I found is that being in the group is a bit like that fear you have standing at the top of a tall building or at the edge of the Grand Canyon. At first you are afraid to even look down (I don't like heights), but gradually you learn to do it and you can see that falling down would be a disaster. Nonetheless you feel better about yourself because you're able to look. that is how I feel about death in the group—I am able to look at it now. I can't say I feel serene, but I can look at it." (Spiegel, 1993b)

HELPER-THERAPY PRINCIPLE

The idea that group members are providing each other with a model for coping with death is another example of the helper-therapy principle applied to this difficult problem. To emerge from a confrontation with such deep anxiety with a sense of pride in being able to help others get through it is no small accomplishment:

A large group meeting was convened by the Wellness Community of Cincinnati to review their program. It consisted of patients with a variety of cancers who participated in support groups, along with their therapists. One slender mother of two young children, there with her husband, spoke up: "I have some bad news that the members of my group here do not yet know. I had a scan yesterday, and there has been a considerable new spread of my disease to my bones and liver. I now realize that this illness is going to shorten my life." There was a stunned silence in the large room, broken by expressions of concern from other group members. "I insisted that my husband and I sit down together last night and plan what is left of my life. We agreed on my will, on funeral arrangements, on care for the children. It may seem hard to believe, but I slept well last night."

The concern in the room was thoroughly leavened by the admiration everyone felt for the forthrightness with which she was handling this sad development in her illness. She had reason to and did feel proud of how she was handling it. She was not denying the need for help in the face of her impending death. In this sense, though dying, she was very much alive and imparting help and meaning to others in showing by example that even the worst news could be borne with dignity and courage.

This response induces more inspiration than dread. She was in no way a bad example of someone giving up in the face of cancer. There are groups in which such a patient would be encouraged not to accept the inevitable, but to psychologically fight the cancer. We have known of patients who have been invited to leave support groups when their cancer recurred, for fear they would demoralize others. This is a terrible mistake. It is not only cruel to the member asked to leave at a time when she needs far more support, but it terrorizes the other members of the group, who now realize that they too will be unacceptable (not just in the group, but in the world at large to the extent that the group models life outside) should they suffer a recurrence. In addition, other members are denied the opportunity to learn from the way in which such members cope with the progression of disease.

Grieving Is Reassuring

Inevitably, the time comes when the anticipation of death is followed by the reality of it. It is no longer just a future fear but a present reality when a group member dies. The notion of grief work was delineated in a classic article written by psychiatrist Eric Lindemann (Lindemann 1944[94]) as a result of his study of reactions to the tragic Coconut Grove nightclub fire. He observed a period of intense restlessness and unhappiness, followed by a time of emotionally burying lost loved ones. He noted that before it could be possible to entertain new relationships, to care about anyone else, it was necessary to grieve losses, to disconnect from loved ones who were gone, to come to terms with their permanent absence while bearing the sadness, helplessness, and anger of their loss. He termed this "grief work." He noted that those few people who initially appeared to bypass this step, acting as though nothing had happened, did far worse in the long run: A number became depressed and were psychiatrically hospitalized years later.

It may seem paradoxical, but in fact there is much reassurance in grieving the loss of someone in the group. Each member experiences the loss of others as their own will be experienced. The more profound her grief and sense of loss, the more she feels in an intensely personal way how much she too will be missed when she dies. The fear of simply disappearing and having life go on unperturbed amplifies death anxiety. The experience of feeling the depth of loss reduces this anxiety.

When one member of the group is dying or dies, it places the other members in the paradoxical position of being the one left behind, rather than the more accustomed role of the one who is dying. This enables them to perceive their dying through the eyes of others:

> The group had been focusing on Caroline, a recent member who had worked her way into the heart of the group quickly through her openness and warmth. She had rapidly progressive disease, and was clearly approaching her death sooner than many other members. Fiona turned to her and said: "You know, I just realized something. I like you but I have been keeping my distance from you, because I know you are dying. I think I have been trying to protect myself from being hurt, from missing you when you die. And now I realize that is what some of my friends and family are doing with me—keeping a distance to avoid being as upset when I die."

When there is a death in a therapy group, it is critical that the full attention of the group be turned to the process of grief work:

> After the death of Eva, a vital and delightful woman who died shortly after a long-planned final trip to Greece, Madeline handed out to the group a series of cards on which she inscribed the following poem, along with a drawing:

> > Dear Eva,

> > Whenever the wind is from the sea
> > salty and strong
> > you are here.

> > Remembering your zest for hilltops
> > and the sturdy surf of your laughter
> > gentles my grief at your going
> > and tempers the thought of my own.

The last two lines capture an important point. Grieving losses of the group strengthens, not weakens, members. This poem became the focus of a discussion about the way in which Eva had faced her death. Often a question by the therapist can stimulate a useful discussion, such as: "What do we miss most about Eva?" Group members admired her strength. She had seen her death coming clearly and had decided to take a final trip before she died. She emphasized being "strong" sometimes at the expense of discussing her weaknesses and concerns openly with the group. They expressed some regret at that. Indeed, they would have preferred to face her death with her directly. They would have welcomed more opportunities to help Eva, and she could have helped them come to terms with her impending death by being even more open about her fears and her resolve to live fully until she died. This underscores the fact that the dying can help the living by giving them a means by which to help the dying face death. This is not usually experienced as a "burden," but rather as an opportunity to do something about their own sense of helplessness and impending loss.

Another useful therapist question in facilitating grieving is, "What is the hardest thing to accept about Eva's death?" The following discussion is typical:

> Shortly after Eva's death, the group members got into a discussion of "giving up the 'escape clause.'" Most had nurtured a secret fantasy that they would be the one to beat the odds. However, as they watched Eva dying, they became increasingly aware of her cancer's relentlessness, and came face to face with a recognition that what they wished had nothing to do with what happened. If that were true in her case, especially given that she was such a vital and determined woman, it must be true in their case as well. Thus their initial admiration of her strength underscored its ultimate limitations, and theirs as well.

Therapists can facilitate discussions such as these and the work of grieving by:

1. using the word "death":

   "I know that Eva's death is very hard for all of us to accept. What has been the most difficult part?"

2. keeping the group focus on the deceased:

   "I know there is concern about other problems, but for the moment, let's keep the focus on Eva's death. We were just talking about . . . "

3. staying with the affect elicited by the loss:

"There seems to be a great deal of sadness in the room. What does it feel like?"

4. encouraging a broadened range of emotional expression, for example, anger as well as sadness:

"Eva elicited many feelings in us. What were some of them?"

5. linking the current loss to past losses in the group, and to future anxieties:

"This is the second loss we have had in six months—that makes it even harder. How does Eva's death feel in the wake of Nancy's?"

In another sense, this process involves anticipatory grief as well. In grieving for others, you are also grieving for yourself, coming closer to a full recognition that the loss will occur, that one's life is not eternal. Death seems inconceivable, and yet when it occurs to others with whom one is close, it becomes more real to oneself as well. Yalom (1980) notes that we come to terms with death in three steps: the impersonal, the interpersonal, and the personal. At first it is just a concept, an abstraction. We know that it occurs even early in life, but death has little personal meaning. However, the death of someone whom we know well and care about brings it into much more intense and personal focus. Thus the grieving of others in the group moves the understanding of death from the impersonal to the interpersonal, and inevitably helps members approach their personal death as well. The ability to grieve for others, a crucial part of the work of such groups, is also reassuring in that the depth of loss is a tangible reminder of each person's own value. In grieving for others, they experience how others will grieve for them.

DOWNWARD COMPARISONS

Cancer patients and those with other life-threatening illnesses have unexpected reactions to disease progression and death in their groups. There is, of course, sadness and fear—empathy by identification. But they also differentiate themselves from those who are dying, and one response does not cancel out the other. The differentiation takes the form of the thought: "We were both dealt the same hand. I am lucky—she is dying and I am still alive. Every day is a gift."

Social psychologist Shelly Taylor (Taylor and Lobel, 1989) has studied support groups of cancer patients, and has observed that they frequently make what she calls "downward comparisons." They find some way to feel better than or luckier than other members of the group. For example, one woman with very advanced disease but a lovely husband will think of another: "I know I am sicker than her, but I wouldn't trade places and have to live with that monster of a husband she is married to." The other woman, healthier but with an admittedly bad marriage, thinks to herself, "I wouldn't trade places with her—I'm not happy with my husband but feel fortunate that I have a chance to live for a while longer."

Thus each woman finds a downward comparison to make with the other, a way to feel lucky despite adverse circumstances. Indeed, when cancer patients compare themselves with others outside such a support group, downward comparisons are much harder to make. In most cases, they are the only obviously ill person—everyone else is feeling sorry for them. However, within the support group, everyone is ill, so in an odd way illness is no longer a defining characteristic. Rather, being ill is taken for granted, and differences among patients are often based on other issues. Furthermore, this allows group members to see their dying on a continuum. The question is no longer being healthy or sick, living or dying. Rather it is living for how long, and how well? This helps group members acquire a different perspective of hope, hope for living longer or better, but not necessarily for escaping the disease entirely.

THE COST OF
NOT FACING DEATH

Much can be lost in the evasion of death.

One young man was planning to quit his job in Washington, D.C., to return to New England where his mother was dying of cancer. However, she had read one of the popular psychology books on cancer that had convinced her that if she just had the right attitude, she did not need to die of the disease. She told him not to quit his job, that she would be fine. At first, her spirits were good, but soon the disease progressed, and she was dead within a year. She and her son lost that last year together because, on the basis of poor advice, they both pretended that she was not dying.

One of the most powerful aspects of group therapy is its role as a laboratory for life, a means of trying out patterns of interaction and receiving feedback about them from other members of the group (Yalom 1995). As group members develop their ability to frankly face and discuss fears of dying and death, they enhance their ability to do the same outside of the group setting.

Rebecca discussed her father's death: "It saddened me that I never really had a chance to talk about my father's dying. It was more upsetting not to know what was really going on. When my father was dying, I kept asking questions and they told me that I asked too many questions." Perhaps it is not accidental that she became a journalist, a profession that more than entitled her to ask questions.

As the ability to talk about the obvious grows, the price of not having done so in the past becomes clearer. The leaders should take every opportunity to pursue discussion of this difficult issue, even if it means putting other things aside. It is fine to say in the midst of an active meeting:

"There are many important issues we could discuss right now, but I think the concern raised by Rebecca and Shirley about what they lost in not being able to discuss their fathers' dying directly is so important that I would like us to pursue it. Has this been the experience of others as well?"

This helps patients to address difficult issues within the group, and also models for them the meaning of helping their families and friends discuss their concerns about their own dying.

The tangible effect that the dying have on the living can be experienced, examined, and evaluated in support groups. It is one thing to talk about how much your family must value your advice, another to give and receive it in the group. The process of drawing a dying person into the center of the group, of valuing her thoughts and feelings, conveys a powerful message about her continued importance. This is a message that the dying need to hear.

BRINGING CONCERNS ABOUT
DEATH TO THE SURFACE

BE DIRECT

The therapist can be helpful by raising questions such as, "I wonder if our difficulty getting going today has to do with the fact that Janet is in the hospital?" Other typical means by which therapists can animate discussion of death and dying involve pursuing predictable but unarticulated consequences of situations that evoke death anxiety. Merely speaking the words often provides greater acceptance of the idea of an open and frank discussion. Psychologist Al Hastorf at Stanford has done research on means by which disabled individuals manage the social discomfort that accompanies their maladies, for example, being in a wheelchair (Hastorf, Wildfogel, et al., 1979). They report that the most effective means of reducing anxiety is to introduce the word *wheelchair* into one of the first few sentences they utter. This is their way of acknowledging what the other person is thinking about, and informing them that they are aware of it and are comfortable enough to discuss it.

Similarly, in the group, the therapist can lead the way by saying, "When your doctor told you that your body was no longer responding to the chemotherapy, you must have been very worried." "Yes," responded the patient, "I thought there was nothing left for him to do." "You thought you were going to die?" asked the therapist. "Of course—if there is nothing left for him to do, and my body is not responding to the medicine, it must mean I'm dying. I couldn't sleep for a week." The therapist asks, "What is the worst part of this fear?"

In this kind of dialogue, the therapist leads the patient a step at a time in the direction of discussing death openly, facing her fears, but also focusing on a particular aspect of her fears as in the last question. In response to such a question, many patients find that it is not so much death as the process of dying that gives them considerable anxiety: fear of losing control over their body, of being in pain, of being unable to make decisions about their treatment, families, and lives. The process of exploring the fear of dying can have the effect of reducing anxiety. Indeed, anxiety can be thought of as a nonspecific sense of discomfort, the intense awareness that something is wrong without certainty about exactly what it is.

It can often be psychotherapeutic to convert the vague awareness of discomfort to something more specific, a fear of something; this starts to circumscribe the anxiety. It also pairs the discomfort with the possibility of responsive action. Anxiety is a kind of "learned helplessness"—there seems to be nothing to do about it. Fear suggests the possibility of protective or restorative action. The sense of being solely in the responsive mode, receiving threats but not acting on them, intensifies anxiety and depression, while having a program of action can reduce it. Thus while there is nothing any of us can do about the threat of nonbeing, there is much to be done about the prospect of diminishing physical ability, increasing pain, treatment choices, and managing relationships. Pursuing the implications of dying to this point suggests not just a proliferation of problems but rather a parsing of them into addressable issues.

EXPECT TO FEEL ANXIOUS

Group leaders should not be alarmed if discussions of mortality make them feel anxious. In fact, leaders should expect to feel anxious. Not experiencing anxiety may be even greater cause for concern. Being aware of their own anxiety about dying suggests that the leaders are fully in touch with their own experience. Clearly, this places them in a better position to help the group members do the same.

The challenge is for the leaders to use their anxiety in a constructive fashion. They may choose to share their internal experience if it seems appropriate, or they may use this self-knowledge to help them be more attuned to what others may be experiencing. Certainly, it is essential that anyone leading these groups be able to tolerate facing their own mortality, since the discussions within the groups raise it in stark form:

Sharon was a trim woman in her fifties with hair cut in a boyish but stylish manner. She was a teacher, the wife of a physician whose practice was eighty miles away. Thus they lived separately during the week. She was proud that she could fend her herself, but it was a strain as well. Her twenty-year-old daughter lived with her but was planning to get a job in San Francisco and move there. Sharon had been having panic-like symptoms, and told the group that she had gotten some bad news: "The cancer seems to be exploding. I have some in my skull—it hurts to comb my hair." She talked tearfully about a nightmare she had recently had: "I awoke from sleep to find a man standing outside the window of my house. I told him to go away and he just leered at me. I tried to call 911 but the phone was dead." She added: "I never have dreams that I can recall, let alone nightmares, so this was particularly striking to me."

The therapist talked about this nightmare as representing "two issues: one clearly is the cancer, in the form of the leering intruder who will not go away, representing the invasion of your body. The second issue in the dream is the inability to communicate." Sharon responded: "Yes, I hadn't thought of it that way, but I wanted someone to rescue me." After further discussion of her fears, the co-therapist said: "We are your 911, and you have been heard." Sharon seemed much comforted by the discussion, and there was a palpable feeling of closeness in the room. The reduced isolation went a long way toward countering Sharon's very palpable death anxiety, compounded by her sense of isolation.

HANDLING NEGATIVE RESPONSES TO DISCUSSING DEATH

It is not uncommon to run across group members who are made anxious by the focus on death and dying. This often arises from a combination of denial, which is challenged, and a mistaken belief that a positive attitude will influence the course of disease.

Christine was feeling rather negative about the group: "Everybody there was talking about dying. People don't need to die of breast cancer. Tell a child it's stupid long enough and it will start to be stupid." The therapist responded: "Well, there is truth to that with children, but it is a more complex matter with cancer." Christine replied, "As a co-dependent [modern jargon for being the partner of an alcoholic] I found it necessary to be able to learn to help others, and I'm good at it." The therapist replied: "I am sure you are. I think it may be harder for you to accept help from others, and this seems like a time when you need it. In my experience, groups like this can be most helpful, even when they are upsetting, if you let others help you."

This idea that contemplating death hastens it, often promulgated in popular alternative health books and the media, makes the kind of realistic support work done in these groups more difficult. Yet such ideas are widespread enough that they must be dealt with from time to time if a direct examination of death and dying is to be carried on. Furthermore, given how emotionally difficult it can be at times to discuss these issues, patients have a right to voice their concerns about the effects of this exploration. Because the path is not easy, members may seek to avoid it. Nonetheless, it is the job of the leaders to look for, explore, and consolidate group discussion of death and dying. Try to cultivate an attitude of realistic hopefulness, balancing an open acceptance of the likely outcome of serious illness with a determination to use the life that remains as richly as possible. Help patients hope for the best but prepare for the worst.

THE PROBLEM OF
ASSISTED SUICIDE

The issue of assisted suicide will inevitably come up in groups of terminally ill patients. Limited legalization of assisted suicide in Oregon has increased awareness of it as an option throughout the country. Many say that they would feel more in control of the remaining portion of their lives if they had a means at their disposal for ending it should it become unbearable or if they felt they had become a burden to their families. However, assisted suicide is often not the solution it appears to be for a variety of reasons.

DEPRESSION

Studies show that 60 percent of those who request assisted suicide meet diagnostic criteria for major depression (Chochinov, Wilson et al., 1995). Suicidal ideation and attempts are common symptoms of depression, and the study cited above makes it clear that depression is the rule, not the exception, among terminally ill patients who request assistance in killing themselves. Any request for assisted suicide should be first considered a sign of depression; the depression should be diagnosed and treated, both with psychotherapy and, if indicated, pharmacologically.

Many factors can affect the competence of a terminally ill patient to decide to die. These include not only depression, but metabolic, infectious, and pharmacological effects of their disease and/or its treatment. Hepatic or renal disease, malnutrition, sepsis, sleep loss, and pain can affect judgment. The usual threshold for competence to consent to medical and surgical procedures is deliberately set quite low: Can patients comprehend the benefits and risks of the procedure? If so, despite even quite severe mental or neurological illness, they are deemed competent. However, a person may well understand the benefits and risks of suicide, yet the decision to proceed with it could be a product of the depression itself, which expresses itself as an undervaluation of the patient's worth to themselves and to their families. Patients often exaggerate the "burden" placed on families by their illness, and have an excessively negative outlook about their illness.

FAMILIES

Two kinds of problems can emerge with families. Often, well-meaning family members think they are being supportive by consenting to pressure from patients: "If it would help you, I will provide the assistance you want." They may do this despite feeling frightened and angry that their wife or other loved one would choose not to be with them, even if for only a few days or weeks. Their consent to help in this manner may in fact confirm fears on the part of the patient that they have become a burden, and that their family would indeed be better off without them. This only falsely reinforces their determination to end their life.

Occasionally there is a more grim scenario in which some families indeed view their ill member as a burden: physical, emotional, or financial. Some may seek to enhance their inheritance by shortcutting the drain on family finances posed by caring for an ill relative. Some vulnerable and dependent patients may well be subjected to pressure to shorten their lives. Such patients must be protected from this kind of pressure.

There is little good research on the long-term effects of having assisted a family member to commit suicide. While it is hard to admit afterwards that such a grave act is a mistake, there is reason to believe that a considerable burden of guilt would accompany a decision to assist a loved one in killing himself or herself. Thus long-term effects on the family should also be considered in evaluating group discussion of assisted suicide.

CURE VERSUS CARE

The modern medical system overvalues cure at the expense of providing adequate care for the dying. In a cure-driven system, both patients and doctors expect that illness will be eliminated rather than coped with, and dying is viewed as a failure rather than a necessary outcome of treating human beings who are mortal. Many patients feel they are "failing" their doctors by getting worse instead of better, and likewise doctors feel they are letting their patients down if they cannot cure them. This has led to avoidance of discussing dying and death, inadequate treatment of pain and suffering in terminal illness, and attention to active "euthanasia" rather than caring. The major hospice organizations are opposed to assisted suicide, because their focus is, appropriately, on compassionate care for the dying. Dying is a natural process, like childbirth, and it deserves the same respect. As one support group patient with advanced breast cancer put it: "Why are we in favor of natural childbirth and artificial death?"

Thus assisted suicide provides no easy answers to the problem of managing dying, and indeed complicates the roles of physicians, nurses, and other health care personnel. When the issue is brought up in groups, it should be addressed openly, not as a quick solution to the problem of dying, but rather as a series of important questions to patients and their families about their value to one another despite a life that is ebbing. Dying should be a means of clarifying ultimate values, rather than dispensing with them.

A group was discussing assisted suicide as a result of Iris's pained description of the increasing limitations placed on her by her disease. "I used to love to see the desert in bloom every spring—now I can barely walk. I'm just becoming a burden. I told my husband I want him to help me end my life when the time comes—soon.

Louanne concurred: "You know it should be like that mask with anesthetic you can get during childbirth. If you get too uncomfortable you put the mask on—if not you can take it off. It's that easy."

"I don't agree," said Jenny. "My aunt hung on for two days, just waiting for me to get there to see her before she died. That time was so precious to me. I know in my heart that she waited for me."

"But she was conscious, you could talk to her, right?" responded Louanne.

"Oh, no. She was in a coma," said Jenny. "But I just know that she was waiting for me to come, and that has always been precious to me."

Sarah, whose religious faith is quite important to her, said: "You know, I believe it is God's decision when we are to die. It is not something we should take into our own hands. We should leave it to Him."

There was much transpiring in this discussion: the ethics of assisted suicide, the meaning of contact with loved ones at the end of life, memories of prior family deaths. The group evidenced considerable disagreement among themselves about these issues. However, they were talking directly about a very difficult topic, and doing it together. They mattered to one another, modeling the importance of the contacts with loved ones that they were discussing. Each was personally drawing from her own life experience to address Iris's question. They treated her as though she mattered very much to them. She was no "burden," but rather deserving of the group's full attention. The process was one of pulling together to examine questions of meaning in life and death. As such it yielded reassurance if not agreement.

Therapists can best deal with this issue openly, by acknowledging deeply held points of view but challenging premature decisions as well. When a patient floats the thought of suicide before the group, it is really a question: "Are you tired of me?" "Would you be better off without me?" It is wise to explore this implicit question with the group, so that their response to the patient is clear. The lack of a response can be interpreted by the patient as a green light. Pursue and clarify the patient's wishes and the reasons for them. Address concomitant issues like pain, disability, and family tensions. Explore how patients can be active about the manner of their death without taking it into their own hands.

CONCLUSION

In each of these examples, the crucial task of the leader has been to direct the discussion toward clear and open confrontation with the threat of death—to look at and beyond it. Avoidance only consolidates the power of the fear and reduces the ability to identify related problems and do something about them. Facing death directly is oddly comforting, especially in a supportive group setting. Including rather than rejecting the dying reassures everyone in the group that they will be cared for throughout their life and death. This discussion demands considerable resilience and clarity of purpose from the group leaders. They must work from a conviction that they are helping rather than hurting group members by asking them to tolerate the discomfort that inevitably comes from a confrontation with death.

CHAPTER 8

Dealing with Isolation, Meaning, and Freedom

Receiving a cancer diagnosis immediately raises questions regarding a person's very existence. Often the first question is, "Am I going to die?" However, along with the concerns regarding death, there are three other existential concerns that routinely arise among patients who have been diagnosed with an illness such as cancer. These concerns have to do with isolation, meaning, and freedom. For example, the question, "Who can possibly understand what I am going through?" speaks to the existential concern of isolation. The question "Why me?" is a clear attempt to make meaning out of the experience and ultimately to find meaning in the universe. "Who am I now that I have cancer?" reflects the existential concern of freedom that comes out of a desire for ground and structure. Here the patient is faced with finding a new ground upon which to reconstruct his or her identity. There are many different kinds of questions or concerns that arise for patients that are existential in nature and consequently strike at the core of the cancer patient's concerns. In the previous chapter, we discussed the existential concerns related to death. In this chapter we focus on isolation, meaning, and freedom.

ISOLATION

There is a way in which each of us is fundamentally alone. We enter the world alone and we will leave alone. No matter how close we get to others, we cannot escape this essential aloneness. Given this ultimate aloneness, there is a striving for connection with others, a longing to close the gap we feel between ourselves and the world. This desire for connection gets expressed in many ways throughout our lives. The desire to merge with a lover, to not die alone, to be looked after, to have someone know the pain we are experiencing—all are expressions of the desire to overcome our existential isolation. "The existential conflict is thus the tension between our awareness of our absolute isolation and our wish for contact, for protection, our wish to be part of a larger whole" (Yalom, 1980, p. 9).

This existential concern is clearly activated by having a life-threatening illness. A diagnosis of cancer removes the person from the mainstream and into a world of confusion, fear, and uncertainty. No longer a part of a familiar and healthy world, the person has suddenly become a patient and has entered a world of disease with an uncertain future. For many there is a sense of being thrust out, on their own, with few around who understand the crisis they are in.

Cancer patients often complain that there are few who understand their experience. To a large extent support groups can counter these feelings but obviously they cannot resolve them. Nevertheless, it is not unusual to hear group members state that they feel less isolated as a result of being in the group. These kinds of statements are another way of acknowledging the wish for contact. The value of group support as an antidote to the chill wind of existential isolation is well described by Yalom in his review of our early experience with cancer support groups (1995).

FACILITATE CONNECTIONS
WITH OTHERS

The terror of having been diagnosed with cancer is exacerbated by the sense of being alone with the physical if not emotional pain of having a potentially life-threatening illness. Who can possibly understand what they are going through? Who *dares* to understand? To understand requires that people face their own existential fears, which most people would rather avoid. Thus, cancer tends to isolate a patient from family and friends. For instance, patients and families often try to spare each other by avoiding difficult topics (Wellisch et al., 1978). Unfortunately, this occurs at a time when the patient needs all the support he or she can get.

The fear that grips cancer patients and the isolation that often ensues can dramatically alter their experience of themselves and the world. Many cancer patients live in terror—a terror that they might not be able to face within themselves or bring themselves to share with others. Sometimes this is because people are unable to listen due to their own fears and anxieties. Sometimes patients feel unable to share their fears because of difficulty in facing the threat to themselves or because of a desire to protect the other person. The end result is the same—isolation and distress. Thus, an important goal of supportive-expressive groups is to improve social support and thereby decrease feelings of isolation.

The following example illustrates how the need for connection remains until the very end and is perhaps intensified as the end draws near. This metastatic breast cancer group was meeting for the first time following the death of a relatively new but much loved member.

Eileen had very quickly worked her way into the hearts of the group members. She had been extraordinarily open for a new member, talking directly about her fears and her desires, about how serious her medical condition was, about the people she cared about in her life. She very quickly came to seem like somebody who had been with the group for a long time.

Members started the meeting reflecting on the fact that she had been there just two weeks ago and had been complaining that she could not drive—and now she was dead. As the group talked it was clear that it frightened them that someone could go so quickly. Then the group shifted to talking about their last encounters with Eileen. Megan talked about being with Eileen the day before she died, that Eileen had been in and out of alertness and for a long time Megan stayed her without her saying very much. But then, after a long silence, Eileen looked at Megan and said, "Megan, you have everything." As Megan relayed this to the group, she smiled her radiant smile and said, "Yes, you know, she was right, I do." Megan went on to talk about how she had come to recognize that what made a relationship valuable was not its length, but what it was like, and that she felt a special kinship with Eileen. Even though her friendship with Eileen had ended very quickly, it had made a difference to her life. Other members also talked about their involvement with Eileen in the days before she died. Several members were moved by how much Eileen wanted to be with them, even within twenty-four hours of her own death. She had let them know that they had touched her and that she wanted them to be a part of her life, even though they had come into it so recently.

As they talked it became clear that Eileen's death was a difficult challenge for the group because it meant facing the worst of their fears. Here was a woman who was upbeat, en-gaging, doing everything she could to live as well as she could, despite the fact that the medical treatments were not retarding the progression of the disease. She was a woman they liked, who they wanted to see more of and have involved in the group. And she had not only died quickly, but rather unpredictably. Thus, while there was some anxiety in the room there was also a sense that they shared a common bond. This sense of being in the same boat was enormously comforting. Even though Eileen ultimately had to suffer and leave this world alone, the women left that night with a sense that neither Eileen nor they were, in fact, completely alone because they still carried Eileen in their hearts.

EMPATHIZE WITH PATIENTS WHO FEEL ISOLATED

The feeling that no one understands what the patient is going through or perhaps that no one cares contributes significantly to the despair that can come out of an awareness of one's existential isolation. An important tool that we have to help patients counter these feelings is empathy. Empathy can be provided by the therapists or it can be given by the group members. The source is less important than the fact that the patient feels his or her experience is both understood and accepted.

Louise had metastatic breast cancer and recently received news that she had four to six months to live. She had a large mass in her liver but, nevertheless, was relieved to learn that she had another week in which to decide whether to have a bone marrow transplant. She described feeling very frightened and alone. She told the group that her sister was irritated with her for postponing the decision about the bone marrow transplant and in-sisted that she had not done enough. This reinforced Louise's sense that people did not understand what she was going through. "I have to trust someone," she said, "and I trust my doctor." The group leader, recognizing that her doctor was running out of "tricks," also saw how much she needed her doctor at this time. He asked her, "I'm won-dering whether you are feeling that your doctor is running out of effective treatment op-tions and that what you need from him right now is to know that he still cares about you." This question spoke to the heart of the matter for Louise and enabled her to talk about how alone she felt knowing that she had so little time.

In another metastatic breast cancer group, Astrid talked about her frustrating efforts to get into an experimental treatment trial. She was initially rejected from the study be-

cause of her poor kidney function, but after much perseverance she managed to talk the
oncologists into putting her into one component of the trial involving gene therapy.
There was a sense of desperation that leaked through as she spoke. Sensing this, the ther-
apist said, "It must be very frightening to find yourself in this place where you have to
search for alternative treatments." This empathic intervention enabled Astrid to access
the terror underneath.

She stated that her feeling was that her options were running out and that the possi-
ble maneuvers to forestall death were becoming fewer and farther between. In addition,
she found three new nodules in her neck and she had some piercing headaches. She said,
"You know I don't talk about this with my family, but it is such a relief to be able to dis-
cuss it here." This discussion led other group members to tell Astrid about their own ex-
periences with aches and pains and their concern that they were due to cancer. Similarly
to Astrid, they found that friends were reluctant to discuss their fears with them, how
it reminds them of their own mortality and so they back away. Hearing the group mem-
bers share their experiences contributed to Astrid's sense of being heard and understood
and was a clear antidote to her being alone in her desperation. It also led to a general dis-
cussion among the members about how caring for one another was a way of dealing with
the feelings of isolation that they feel facing death and the limitations imposed on them
by the illness.

MEANING

"If we must die, if we constitute our own world, if each is ultimately alone
in an indifferent universe, then what meaning does life have? . . . The existential dynamic conflict stems from the dilemma of a meaning-seeking crea-
ture who is thrown into a universe that has no meaning" (Yalom, 1980, p. 9).
Although some might disagree that the universe has no meaning, there is no
denying that we have a need to make meaning out of our lives. There is also
no denying that we continually make choices about how to live our lives
and how to make sense of ourselves and the world.

Although the need to make meaning is ever present, there are times when
this need is more acute, such as during adolescence, during a midlife crisis,
or when someone has been diagnosed with a serious disease. A diagnosis of
cancer accentuates the existential concerns with meaninglessness. Consequently, patients are often preoccupied with such questions as, Why did I
get the disease? or What do I want to do with my life now that I have cancer? As a result, life priorities are often reevaluated.

WHY ME?

The question "Why me?" is frequently heard among patients newly diagnosed with cancer. It is a clear and poignant expression of the need to make sense out of meaninglessness. For most patients, the question usually refers to whether there was something they did or did not do that caused the cancer to occur. Was it the food they ate, the stress they were under, a genetic disposition, or because of where they live? Perhaps what is most frightening about getting cancer is the thought that it is random and hence unpredictable. The question "why" suggests that they could have done something to prevent the disease or that they can now do something to impede its progress. Living with the knowledge that there is no definitive answer to this question leaves the patient with the profound discomfort that comes from living in a meaningless universe.

> Bernice had been recently diagnosed with primary breast cancer. During her group meeting she stated that she was feeling confused and frightened and that she was shocked by what she'd gone through. "It's as though I can't believe that this is happening to me or why it's happening." She found that she was now in a constant state of dread, waiting for something to go wrong. She even worried that her dog would die. She also cried at the smallest things, such as her cat eating the house mouse. She questioned why she has had to fight so hard in her life. "When is this calamity going to stop? I'm tired of being the hero and then getting the short end of the stick. I'm sick of it and want it to stop."
>
> Bernice also wondered why she was feeling this way now because she didn't feel anywhere near this bad when she was going through treatment. She should be feeling better but is feeling worse. The therapist remarked that her reactions are not uncommon. "Could it be," she asked, "that when you were going through chemo you were doing something about the cancer and that gave you a sense of control over the illness? Now you are faced again with your feelings of helplessness and lack of control." Bernice then asked, "How do you express to people that the problems now are so profoundly psychological?"

This was an important question that reflected the isolation patients experience by having their existential concerns rise to the surface. It also illustrates that existential concerns are often interconnected and that an awareness of one concern (in this case, meaninglessness) often activates another (e.g., isolation).

HELP PATIENTS REORDER PRIORITIES

A frank discussion about death provides the occasion for better planning of the life that remains. One of the cruelest things to do to someone with a shortened life expectancy is to pretend that it is longer than it is. The sense of realistic urgency that comes with impending death can mobilize people to do the things that matter.

> *One woman who was dying of breast cancer talked about how the tragedy of her mother's death from breast cancer was compounded by her unwillingness to talk about it: "We could never discuss it. We knew she was dying, and she did, but we could not talk about it. I wish I had said more to her, and she had said more to me. Now I tell my family how much I love them—still not often enough—but I am determined not to make the same mistake my mother did."*

The awareness of needing to take advantage of whatever time is left can be activated directly by events that unfold in the life of the group. For example, in our metastatic breast cancer groups, where there have been numerous deaths, many of our group members have become painfully aware of lost opportunities and have resolved to use their time differently in the groups. In one group, two members died within days of each other. One death was expected and the other was not. The unexpected death stirred up a good deal of feeling, particularly feelings of incompleteness because the survivors had not been able to say good-bye. While this raised concerns for what had been lost, it also raised questions regarding what to do in the future. Megan raised the question beautifully: "What are the things we should say to each other before it is too late?" This led the group into heartfelt expressions of love and caring for one another. Each member left that meeting knowing that they had shared their most important feelings with each other.

Therapists can help facilitate the discussion of reordered priorities by addressing the meaning of the limitation on time that impending death imposes. "Given the limitations that you are facing, what matters most to you now? What do you want to be sure you accomplish? What kind of a legacy do you want to leave?" One woman answered this question by creating a journalism scholarship in her name. This was her way of ensuring that she made a lasting contribution to the field she so dearly loved. Another option for therapists is to ask others in the group how they have changed their use of time in the face of their illness. Clarifying priorities and expectations of others is one of the few advantages of having a potentially life-threatening illness.

Patients will often express their frustration over wasted time. This can take the form of complaining about obligations that feel more like a burden than anything else. Helping patients recognize that their time is precious naturally leads them into reorganizing their priorities.

> Group members are usually the first to encourage someone to let go of unimportant obligations. Such was the case when one woman talked about the spring cleaning she needed to do and how this was preventing her from going away for the weekend. This was met with a chorus of amazement that she would even have a doubt about what she should do. "Hire a house cleaner," said one woman. "So what if your windows are dirty," said another." "The dirt will be there when you get back but this opportunity to get away with your husband will be lost," said a third. It didn't take too long for her to realize what was a more valuable use of her time.

DRAW PATIENTS OUT OF SELF-ABSORPTION

Death is infinite and overwhelming. The proximity of it can be like a whirlpool, drawing into it all thoughts that come near. This can suck the meaning out of life, making the person feel already lifeless, what Kierkegaard called the "sickness unto death" (Kierkegaard, 1954), feeling dead while alive, devoid of spontaneity, choice, and meaning. Conversely, anything that affirms your life force, meaning, and importance to others counters this sense that death has already claimed you. Yalom (1995) describes this process in cancer support groups:

> For one thing, the members were deeply supportive to one another, and it was extraordinarily helpful for them to be so. Offering help so as to receive it in reciprocal fashion was only one, and not the most important, aspect of the benefits to be gained. Being useful to someone else drew them out of morbid self-absorption and provided them with a sense of purpose and meaning. Almost every terminally ill person I have spoken to has expressed deep fear of a helpless immobility—not only of being a burden to others and being unable to care for themselves but of being useless and without value to others. Living, then, becomes reduced to pointless survival, and the individual searches within, ever more deeply, for meaning. The group offered these patients the opportunity to find meaning outside themselves: by extending help to another person, by caring for others, they find the sense of purpose that so often eludes sheer introspective reflection. (p. 95)

Thus, the tangible sense of having meaning to others counters death anxiety by underscoring the person's continued vitality and interpersonal importance: "I may be dying, but I'm not dead yet."

Corinne was a single mom with metastatic breast cancer who tended to feel very sorry for herself. She also had reason to. No one could deny that she was in a difficult and painful situation. Her cancer was progressing, she couldn't bear to tell her young daughter about how serious her illness was, and she was alone. Consequently, she usually spent her time in group talking about her problems. While she claimed that the group support was helpful to her, she also seemed caught in the trap of her own problems. One day Stella, another group member, informed the group that she had just learned from her oncologist that her cancer had progressed. Stella's situation was also not good and yet she managed to be quite matter-of-fact about her situation. Stella had always been very supportive of Corinne, and Corinne clearly was taken aback by Stella's news.

After Stella had described her situation, Corinne talked openly about her fears for Stella, who was being stiff-upper-lipped about her situation. Stella said rather brusquely, "You're just worried about yourself." Clearly, Stella was attempting to push Corinne away because Corinne was moving into a sensitive area for Stella. Corinne held her ground and responded, "Well, that's true, but I am also worried about you." The therapist asked Corinne, "Can you tell us what you are worried about?" This question enabled Corinne to tell Stella about her concerns that Stella is closing herself off emotionally out of fear and that it was time she allowed someone to support her. This initiated an extremely helpful discussion that was focused on Stella. By the end of the session not only had Stella expressed both her fear about the disease progression and her gratitude for the group support, Corinne also appeared completely buoyed by the experience. For a change, she was the one giving support, and ironically this appeared to have helped her more than anything else.

Suicide is perhaps the ultimate expression of the concern with meaninglessness. It also most clearly demonstrates self-absorption. Thus, drawing suicidal patients out of their self-absorption is a primary goal. Suicide was the topic of discussion in one of our metastatic breast cancer groups. There was a clear division in the group, with two members advocating their right to commit suicide and the rest of the group urging them to consider the effect of suicide on others.

Iris stated that she wanted suicide as an option in case her situation gets too bad. She wondered aloud about how a person gets information on how to do it. Louanne re-

sponded that she had the means to do it. At this point the therapist asked Louanne what she was afraid of. She said that she had always been healthy and was afraid of being remembered by her family as having been sickly. To this Iris also responded that she wanted to protect her family from seeing her suffer and she did not want the last memory of her to be her dying a painful death.

On hearing their reasons, the group members urged these women to think about the effect that their suicide would have on the people who care about them. Rather than protecting their families, they argued, they would be hurting them. One woman talked movingly about the circumstances of her husband's suicide 30 years earlier and its lingering effects on her and their children. Another woman spoke about the death of her mother from a long illness and how she treasures the last days she had with her. Rather than being left with a haunting memory, she remembers the love they expressed to each other in those final days. While this discussion did not immediately change the minds of Iris and Luanne, it was the beginning of an ongoing dialogue in the group regarding suicide and responsibility to others.

FREEDOM

The existential concern of freedom is about living with the absence of structure. Although we generally think of freedom as a positive concept, from an existential viewpoint it is linked to the experience of dread. Dread arises because having freedom to choose how we live, in having to "create" our lives, implies that underneath all that we have created for ourselves there is a void. Thus, the existential conflict is "the clash between our confrontation with groundlessness and our wish for ground and structure" (Yalom, 1980, p. 9). Common ways in which concerns regarding freedom are expressed include concerns of identity, making choices, and lack of control.

HELP PATIENTS REDEFINE THEMSELVES

One predictable consequence of having cancer is that it challenges the patient's identity. The challenge to the patient's identity occurs on many levels—physically, emotionally, psychologically, interpersonally. Cancer has a way of disrupting the sense of self that the patient has constructed, thereby demanding a reconstruction. For instance, at a purely physical level patients are faced with having their bodies mutilated and scarred, their energy sapped, and/or a loss of some or even all of their hair. This leaves patients feeling that their bodies are no longer familiar. Yet, somehow, they must find a way to claim these transformed bodies as their own.

Diane was a thirty-four-year-old woman who had a mastectomy after being diagnosed with primary breast cancer. She was ten months postsurgery and was having difficulty resuming sexual relations with her husband. Diane cried as she told the group about how she could barely look at herself in the mirror. If she can't look at herself, how can she ever be comfortable with herself sexually again, she lamented. She described feeling mutilated since her mastectomy and ashamed to let her husband see her scar. The despair and hopelessness that Diane expressed was familiar to many of the group members. The therapist, sensing that Diane would benefit from learning how others overcame such feelings asked, "How have others in the group handled this kind of issue?" Drawing on the experiences of other women helped normalize the situation for Diane. Hearing others describe similar concerns about being sexually desirable, and how they overcame it, was deeply reassuring. By hearing about the process that each of them went through in reclaiming their bodies, she realized that she too needed to find a way to make her body acceptable to herself.

In another group of metastatic breast cancer patients, Rebecca reported that she had been quite depressed and that the deaths of Jane and Rita had really gotten to her. Even her husband had noticed a difference. However, she also felt that her husband had been more remote and not available to her. When the therapist asked what she meant, she said, "Well, when I start talking about how depressed I am, he says, 'Look, I'm sad about this too.'" The group reflected back to her that this didn't sound like he was unwilling to talk with her. Stella recalled the time she had been out with Rebecca and her husband and how he certainly seemed to love her very much. Then Rebecca said, "But what's to love? He married an ambitious, smart, witty, hard-working person, and what am I now?" The real issue seemed to be her despair over her dismantled identity.

Several of the women commiserated with Rebecca on how they too felt that their sense of self had been irrevocably altered. At the end of the discussion, Rebecca said that she felt better, that she felt understood, and did not feel as depressed, having talked about what was depressing her. One touching moment near the end of the session occurred when Rebecca said, "You know, I've lost all of these things, this wittiness, the sharp edge. Now I feel all amorphous and fuzzy." "That's wonderful," Megan said with a big smile on her face. It was a touching moment in which Megan suddenly restructured Rebecca's loss into the idea that a new and valuable part of herself was emerging.

ORPHEUS EXERCISE

One method we use to facilitate an examination of a changed identity is the Orpheus exercise, developed by existential psychologist James Bugental (1973–1974). Bugental named the exercise after this tragic figure in Greek mythology because Orpheus symbolizes resistance to accepting loss. The story is that Orpheus, in despair over the death of his bride, Eurydice, descended into Hades to plead for her release. The gods took pity on him and released her on one condition—Orpheus was not to look behind to see her until they had ascended to Earth. However, in a moment of weakness he stole a glance backward, and Eurydice was gone forever. Orpheus symbolizes resistance to accepting loss because acceptance requires leaving what has been left behind and looking ahead.

First we briefly explain the purpose of the exercise and then ask members to close their eyes and mentally to make a list of attributes, aspects of themselves, that have been important to them—for example, teacher, mother, hiker, skier, cook, journalist. Then they are asked to rank these aspects of themselves, from least to most central to their sense of personal identity. Once they have done this we ask them to imagine giving each one up, starting with the least important one: "Ask yourself this question: 'Who am I if I am no longer this?'"

This exercise elicits substantial emotion, since the losses they are grappling with are often real and not theoretical. Their illness often forces people to give up long-cherished aspects of themselves.

After a few moments, ask the group to open their eyes and discuss the loss of the first attribute. As the discussion progresses, ask the group to close their eyes again and imagine giving up the second attribute on the list, moving closer to the core, and again ask the question "Who am I?" As they move closer to the core, feelings will run even stronger.

Raina spoke movingly about her sadness in no longer being a long distance runner. Accepting her radically altered body and depleted energy was one of the more difficult adjustments she had had to make. However, as she considered the question of "who am I now that I no longer run?" she discovered that she had learned to become a grandmother. Because she no longer spent so much of her time training for marathons, she now had time to spend with her grandchildren and she realized what a great joy this had become to her. By losing a part of herself that had been so central to her indentity and that had consumed so much of her time, Raina came to discover parts of herself that she had given little attention to or opportunity for expression. She realized how grateful she was for this unexpected gift.

As they picture each aspect of their identity being stripped away and as they get closer to the core of their being, patients often become clearer about what is most important to them and also how to use that knowledge to make better choices. We tend to lose ourselves in our roles, making us more like a thing, a collection of attributes. The process of giving up old roles and taking on new ones puts us back in touch with the deeper truth about ourselves (Kierkegaard, 1954).

Encourage Responsibility to Others

Out of the conflict between groundlessness and the desire for ground and structure comes the responsibility to create our lives. It is up to us to choose how to live our lives. As cancer patients are faced with the crumbling of the worlds they had previously constructed, they now have the responsibility to re-create their lives. The role of the therapist is to help patients recognize the choices they are making and that there are times when patients need to take into account their responsibility to others.

It is easy to become so absorbed in the despair surrounding the illness that patients overlook their ongoing responsibilities to others. This is bad for everyone, making the ill person feel more isolated, and depriving others of what they need. Sometimes this withdrawal is aided and abetted by well-meaning but misinformed family members.

In one group meeting, a woman with metastatic breast cancer who had young children told the group how enraged she became when she overheard her husband saying to her nine-year-old son: "Don't bother Mommy with your homework—I'll help you later." "Look," she said to her husband, "I can't do much anymore. I can't cook. I can't clean. I can't work. But one thing I can do is help my child with his homework." The husband, thinking he was protecting his wife, was in fact depriving her of opportunities to nurture her children.

When patients are very ill and death is approaching, it is important to help them see that they still have choices to make regarding how to live the

remaining life. Although the following example did not take place in a support group, it demonstrates how therapists can help patients recognize their
responsibility to others and therefore help them make better choices for the
time that is left.

> One morning, a psychiatrist was called to handle an emergency in the oncology clinic.
> An older gentleman, who was within weeks of death from lung cancer, had tried to jump
> to his death out of his second-story bedroom window. When the psychiatrist arrived he
> was sitting in a wheelchair with head bowed, surrounded by his tearful family: wife,
> children, and in-laws. He had no prior history of depression, psychiatric treatment, or
> suicidal ideation. "What is going on?" the psychiatrist asked. "I'm no use to any of
> them. I'm just a burden. They would be better off without me," he said quietly. Hearing
> this, his wife cried harder. "I wonder if you are not overlooking something," the psychi-
> atrist said. He looked up and asked, "What?" "Every one of these people in your family
> standing around you will die someday. You are still the head of the family. You have a
> responsibility to provide them with a model for how to die. At the moment, frankly, you
> are doing a lousy job of it."
>
> There was a long pause, during which the referring oncologist seemed to have second
> thoughts about the consultation. However, after a few minutes, the frail, elderly gentle-
> man called his son-in-law over and said: "You know that air conditioner in my room
> doesn't work and it is hot up there. I want you to get it fixed." This directive to his son-
> in-law showed that this man had chosen to resume his role as head of the family. Choos-
> ing to define his current existence as head of the household, in spite of the fact that he
> was dying, gave his remaining days a greater sense of meaning and enabled him to re-
> main connected to his family. He died peacefully of the cancer several weeks later.

ENCOURAGE LIVING FULLY
IN THE PRESENT

We encourage patients to live fully in the present and we help them to recognize that this is a choice they have. We accomplish this by making the present
moment a focus of our groups. Thus, we are always attending to affective experience and group process. When feelings come up for people, we inquire
after them and help patients to be rooted in the "here-and-now" by sharing
their experience with the group. If something seems to have been communicated nonverbally among the group members, we will encourage members
to give words to their feelings. For instance, if group members rally around a
member who is in need of support by offering advice and suggestions, the
group leader might comment on the concern and caring that is being shown

to that person. The aim is to help patients learn to be aware of their ongoing experience and to make conscious choices about what to do about that experience, such as whether to express one's feelings to another.

Some people have a far greater difficulty both accessing their here-and-now experience and making conscious choices about that experience. The group can be helpful in both modeling and encouraging the group member.

Bernice was usually quite reserved but in this meeting was far more talkative than usual. She told the group that it used to be that when she started to cry, her husband would tell her not to cry and then she would be all right. When the group leader asked how she felt about that, she said, "I wanted to slug him." She also talked about how her husband wanted to come with her to her oncologist. She had an appointment that afternoon, at which time a decision would be made about whether she had to resume chemotherapy. She said she didn't want her husband there because he tended to take over. At this point, one member pointed out that some husbands may need that sense of reassurance by being in touch with the oncologist themselves.

Because Bernice had not received an empathic response to a rare moment where she had expressed her inner feelings, the therapist was concerned that it might have the effect of further shutting Bernice down. In an attempt to support Bernice and help her talk about her reaction to the feedback, the therapist asked her what it was like to get this response. "It's fine," she replied. Because it did not feel "fine" to the therapist, the therapist suspected it did not feel fine to Bernice either. The therapist persisted saying, "Your story about your husband responding to your crying by telling you not to cry suggested to me that it can be upsetting to not have your feelings acknowledged. At the same time it also seems that you often keep your feelings to yourself. I'm wondering if you are doing that right now." This intervention opened the door to Bernice acknowledging her true feelings and finally getting the support she needed.

WORKING WITH EXISTENTIAL CONCERNS IN THE CONTEXT OF RELIGIOUS BELIEFS

Clearly, work with cancer patients, many of whom are actively dealing with dying and death, approaches a domain traditionally occupied by various religious beliefs and religious traditions. These groups are not meant to replace, challenge, or discount members' religious faith. On the other hand, they are not a place for recruiting others to a given religious belief. They are meant to help people to better manage the process of both living and dying, rather than to explain to them the meaning of life and death and their place in the universe.

For some, their place after death is clearly defined by their religious beliefs; others are quite certain that they live in a random universe and that the problems of existence will be left to their family and friends after their death. Some are unsure. Death and beyond, while faced in these groups, are not explained in them. This approach is profoundly respectful of religious tradition, but also different from it.

CONCLUSION

While we all are faced with resolving our existential concerns, this challenge comes to the fore when living with cancer. In this chapter we illustrate some of the ways in which these existential concerns can be expressed in group and we provide some guidelines for facilitating an examination of these issues. These existential concerns are oftentimes so interconnected that they are difficult to separate. In those cases, we recommend helping the group members to identify their most pressing concern.

Usually there are few places where patients can address fundamental concerns about their existence. This may be one reason our groups have been described by some of our members as a "sanctuary." An avowed atheist in one of our groups described the group as her "church." Perhaps this is because these groups are a place to talk about ultimate concerns.

PART FOUR
MANAGING GROUP PROBLEMS
AND SPECIAL SITUATIONS

CHAPTER 9

Facilitating Family and Specialized Groups

FAMILY GROUPS

The family is itself a natural grouping, the primordial source of support. Nonetheless, at times of serious threat and disruption, family members may benefit from additional support in the form of groups for family members. Family members desperately cling to the hope of keeping everything the same even as cancer constitutes a major life and family change. This seems a way of yielding the minimum necessary to the illness, to maintain as much as possible of what has been good in life. Yet the illness does exact a toll and requires accomodation within families. Family groups are a useful means of exploring these changes.

FAMILY GROUPS WITH OR WITHOUT THE PATIENT

Although we have run family groups with and without patients, we favor those with the family members alone for the following reasons:

1. In such groups, the family members are the ones with the problem. Cancer or other life-threatening illness is such a serious challenge that anyone else's difficulties often seem trivial by comparison. Thus there is a sense in which the cancer patient's problems always trump

those of the spouse or child: she is the one with the serious illness. Yet those are the very same problems confronting family members: frustration, fear, anger, helplessness; these problems must be addressed in a group because they are so often put in second place at home. Family members commonly feel that they do not "deserve" to have concerns because those of the ill family member are so much more serious. In a support group composed solely of family members, these "second-ranking" problems are by definition the heart of the discussion. As one husband of a breast cancer patient put it, "This group is a place where I come to feel better about feeling bad."

2. Having cancer patients in one group of their own and family members in another suggests the differences in their problems and their capacities to do things separately. For example, husbands have used family groups to come to terms with the idea that they are likely to outlive their spouses. As they watch others go through this process, the future loss becomes real to them. They can contemplate planning for life beyond the loss of their loved one, and though it is a terrible thing to go through, others are able to get through it. The reality of potential loss is brought home in such groups, as is the possibility of navigating one's way through it. Participation in family groups can thus help to facilitate the grieving process through anticipatory grieving. In fact, to participate in a group that does not include the ill family member is a trial experience of life without that person.

3. Separate groups provide the patient and the family with an opportunity to debrief each other about what happened in their respective groups, thereby stimulating discussion about common problems. Thus, the need to convey what transpired in each group can actually be a stimulus to further communication between patient and family. Of course, issues of confidentiality are important. Be sure to have a discussion with each of your groups regarding what rules they want to establish about what can and cannot be shared outside of group.

4. Such a grouping respects the privacy of communication within couples, allowing them to settle personal disagreements and discuss problems on their own.

Nevertheless, there are obvious advantages to groups involving both patients and their families. Such groups can work more effectively on interaction patterns between patient and family. Difficulties in communicating needs and working out means of supporting one another can be more directly addressed. Families can model for one another means of clarifying communication and providing support. They can also provide feedback to one another about their communication. In our experience, feedback is usually far more effective when it comes from the members than when it comes from therapists. Sometimes family members get stuck in their communication patterns and it can be helpful to hear the perspective of someone outside the family who also understands the difficulties they face.

Couples in which one of the partners has cancer have special problems, which separate them from others who are not dealing with cancer. In a sense the couple carries the disease with them, since the illness affects the whole family, not just the patient. Their difficulties as couples in dealing with "normal" healthy families can be addressed. In this respect, it can be extremely helpful to hear about the experiences of other couples who are in similar circumstances. How have they dealt with the stigma attached to having cancer or the ways in which they have been treated differently?

In both types of groups, members can fulfill "as if" roles, providing feedback about what a parent or a partner might feel based on their own experience. This allows for a knowledgeable but dispassionate view about the difficulties inherent in living with serious illness.

GENERAL PRINCIPLES

Group Size.   Twelve people is usually the upper size limit for a manageable psychotherapy group. Since there may be several members from each family—husband, wife, older children, parents, brothers, or sisters—it might be important to limit the number of members per family. When appropriate we also define "family" loosely and allow close friends of patients to participate. There is value in the opportunity to witness the problems of others as a sympathetic outsider and to note how other families cope with similar difficulties. To do this, there needs to be room for a variety of families to participate. Fortunately, we have not had to refuse any members from joining a family group.

Introducing Group Members.   Family groups can be quite varied in terms of age, gender, health status, and life circumstances. Ask members to introduce themselves and to tell a little bit about the person in their family who has cancer (presuming that this is the type of group in which those with cancer do not participate). These initial stories should be enough to establish the common ground among group members but not be a long and detailed review of their loved one's medical history.

This initial introduction also serves to help everyone feel that they have an equal right to the floor, that their problems are as worthy of examination by the group as anyone else's. It is crucial that everyone feel as much a part of the group as possible. When new members join the group, ask them to briefly describe their situation, thereby establishing their credentials. For example, "I'd like to introduce Steve and his daughter Randi and welcome you to the group. Could you tell us a little about what brings you here?"

Some family members may be reticent to speak right away. They may be accommodated in the following way: "Welcome to the group. Some new members like to wait a little while to get the lay of the land before telling us a little about themselves. Others prefer to introduce themselves right away. What would you like to do?"

This establishes the expectation for the new members and the group that they will talk about their experience with a loved one who has cancer at some point during the meeting, but allows them some time to prepare if they wish to have it.

Assessing Critical Issues. It is crucial that the hard things be talked about. The therapists should be assessing throughout the meeting what are the most difficult and important issues, and bring them to the center of the discussion. Indications of the importance of issues include:

1. Signs of visible emotion—tears, sadness, anxiety, anger;
2. The effect of the threatened or actual death of a loved one on family members;
3. Difficulties in caring for a loved one who is ill;
4. Communication problems within families;
5. How to provide support to a family member who is ill;
6. Effects of the loved one's illness on the family; and
7. Discomfort or tensions among group members.

The therapists' task, both during the initial meeting and in regular meetings, is to scan the group and the discussion for relevant emotion and content, and to bring them to the group's attention. The important themes will be similar to those in a group of patients with the illness, yet there will be crucial differences: the frustrations of a physically healthy family member accepting the effects of disease and its treatment on a loved one, the forced changes in family life imposed by the illness, the need to abandon old roles and take on new ones.

In a well-functioning group there may well be more than one salient issue vying for attention. Any one may be a good starting point. But there will also be distracting issues: comparing medical treatments, advocating fringe remedies, discussion of job, school, or unrelated financial problems. The therapist needs to make a decision about the salient material and reinforce it. It is particularly helpful to begin thinking about common themes across the problems presented. The leader may notice, for example, that several members have begun discussing their sense of helplessness in responding to the symptoms produced by the illness. The therapist might say, "I notice that several of you have brought up situations that are difficult for your loved one and which leave you feeling helpless. I wonder if we could talk about that sense of helplessness." Here the problem is brought up without any suggestion of an immediate resolution—that will come later.

If there is a lot going on and the common theme is not obvious, it can be quite useful to articulate the therapist's dilemma: "I realize that we have a number of important issues to deal with, and we probably can't do justice to all of them. John, you seem upset—shall we start with you?" This conveys to the group that other hot topics are equally important, but the therapist wants to move the group in the direction of problems involving the illness and its effects on families, particularly those that stir up strong feelings.

Keeping Involvement Balanced.   There is no such thing as equal time in groups. Some members by nature or by dint of their immediate problems will talk more than others. However, it is crucial that everyone feel involved, at least potentially if not actually. All members should feel that they could participate if they wanted to. They should be listening actively, rather than just waiting their turn. If one or more members seems detached from the discussion, find a moment to ask them about it: "John, you seem a bit distracted. Is this discussion hard for you to relate to?"

These groups are complicated by the family dynamics that are inherent in their structure. Children may be reticent to discuss certain issues with their father in the room, or may feel that their father should set the stage by raising an issue before they elaborate upon it. There is concern in such a situation of airing dirty laundry in public, and the therapist can facilitate greater openness by asking other members of the same family to comment on their reactions to what they have just heard before opening discussion to the wider group. This invites fuller participation from the family and increases the richness of the presentation of the problem.

One group was discussing how much to share their own fears and emotional response with the patient.

> Sharon's mother said: "I try to keep in control with Sharon and go home and close the door and cry." The therapist raised questions about this strategy. Gretchen's sister, who was pregnant, said that she feels reluctant to bring up her happiness, given how sick her sister is, and added "I feel somewhat guilty about sharing too much of this happiness with her. At the same time, I'm afraid. My sister was thirty-four when she got cancer. I am about to turn thirty-four." The therapist noted that this fear was something she had not shared with Gretchen, and that her sister was quite expert in dealing with it. Sharing that might make it easier to share her happier moments as well, because she would be less different from her sister in discussing their common fears as well. By sharing their reluctance to discuss their own fears, they came to acknowledge their common situation, felt more open and closer with one another, and developed a strategy for opening up their communication with ill family members.

Acknowledging and Summarizing Before Moving On.   There is no number of issues that can be dealt with in a given group. Usually in ninety minutes, one to three major themes can be addressed adequately. A therapist can often feel when an issue has been adequately dealt with and when it is time to move on: The emotional tone loses intensity, the discussion becomes a bit repetitive, a key issue has been dealt with and resolved. A good transition involves acknowledging and summarizing what has just transpired so that the direction is not experienced as a negation or dismissal of what has previously been discussed. Indeed, even apparently disparate themes usually complement one another:

> Laurie's family commented that they were upset that Laurie seemed somewhat "closed down," not open to their suggestions. At the same time, her father spoke in a rather dry manner, and focused on finding some alternative treatments for his daughter. He was convinced he could change the course of her breast cancer progression: "What is, was." The therapist commented on the difficulty people have in accepting the hard realities of illness. Alison's friend commented that there were times when "Alison simply does not wish to be prodded into some kind of intense interaction, so I just sit with her."

Several husbands then shifted the discussion to their own difficulty in accepting an un-pleasant reality that "just has to be dealt with from time to time but not all the time." Thus they began to focus more on their own sense of helplessness and away from the family member's withdrawal or recalcitrance. Rather than fix it, they started to feel some of the same helplessness that the patient must be feeling, and learn to tolerate that feeling, albeit "not all the time."

Summarizing the Main Theme or Themes at the End of the Group.   It is helpful for the therapist to review the major issues or themes that have been discussed at the end of the meeting. This review helps to consolidate what has come from the family group. The experience, as noted in Chapter 6, is meant to be more than catharsis. The meaning extracted from often difficult and emotional discussion should be underscored and summarized.

As the group just described came to an end, several members commented that they often thought about what others had said during the period between groups and that it meant a great deal to them. They also said that they were deeply affected by upsetting news about members. The therapist commented that being able to tolerate the feeling of help-lessness that comes with seeing family members being so ill is hard, but it also can bring people closer to those who are experiencing the same helplessness because of their own illness.

This discussion acknowledged the emotional difficulty of the group work, and also underscored its benefits—facing directly what lay ahead and seeing that there are ways to cope.

MAJOR THEMES IN FAMILY GROUPS

The major themes in family groups reflect and build upon themes in the supportive-expressive groups for those with cancer.

Building Bonds.   Just as cancer patients feel very alone with their illness, their families also feel immersed in a situation that burdens them and in which they can expect little in the way of support from others. Like cancer patients, they often find that friends are helpful at first, but quickly tire of the sustained misery that chronic and progressive illness can bring. Family groups provide a context for establishing a common ground, a sense of being in a situation that is difficult but not unique.

Kelly's husband, a new group member, started talking about the pressures he had been under with his wife's illness. He added that he had been in AA and had been "clean and sober" for three years. He started banging on the chair and yelling: "I can't stand the thought of losing Kelly." The therapist, in a voice intended to impose calm but also acknowledge his concerns, asked him to describe more about the thought of losing Kelly. "I have to push her to make dinner now. She wouldn't be happy if I didn't get her to do it."

It became clear that Kelly's husband was more worried about his loss of supportive resources than her illness. Such revelations can be difficult moments.

Jake, another husband, seemed quite upset, and said: "My wife's ups and downs really get to me." Carl added, "I simply hope for the best. I can't even think that my Nancy is getting worse." Several others talked about their reaction to the potential loss of their wives. Michael said: "Well, you finally did it, you brought up the 'D' word."

The price of being "strong" in reaction to the potential loss of their wives was that it separated them from their wives. Managing these feelings of loss was difficult and involved acknowledging how bad things might get. This group interaction started out with an almost embarrassing display of the primary fear of loss of support. Yet it was honest—these husbands had good reason to fear the loss of support. In varied and more modulated form, others admitted to similar concerns, thereby normalizing their reactions. Expressing these feelings gave them a sense of commonality, and built a sense of belonging in the group.

Rick and Ron talked about the first Christmas without their wives—how they had struggled to make things the same and yet different. They knew that they would get through. Rick fought back tears as he talked about writing the Christmas letter without his wife editing it and filling out the addresses. Now he felt good that he had gotten through it. The therapist asked, "Has anyone else had that feeling at holiday time?"

Jamie, the daughter of a woman with breast cancer, then tearfully related how she had come home expecting to have the intensity that her mother had tried to induce the previous year, when she thought it would be her last Christmas. Her father told her that this year it would be different because they had been preoccupied with a move. She saw her mother as counting each year, each Christmas that passed, not as one more but as one less that lay ahead. Then another group member suggested that perhaps her mother

had sensed that the intensity had been too hard on her, and had deliberately reduced the
emotional intensity of the family holiday.

The theme of commonality was reinforced by a discussion of how the group seemed to be a kind of road map of what lay ahead. Experiences that were intensely personal were also found to be common among group members. Thus the distress they felt cemented the bonds of shared experience and understanding among group members.

Sharing Emotion.   As in the groups for cancer patients, expression of strong feeling is encouraged. The leaders' task is to look for signs of strong feelings and pull for exploration of them.

> *Isabel began to cry as she talked about how painful it was to think about being without*
> *her mother. She had images of her lying on the floor, unable to call anyone to help her.*
> *She talked about long phone calls they had when they cried together, and how she felt*
> *she was being a burden to her mother rather than a help.*

This juxtaposition of expressed emotion and concerns about its effects at home is a golden opportunity for the therapist to use the group interaction to provide an immediate and powerful response to Isabel's concern.

> *The therapist asked, "Let me interrupt and ask the group at this point how it feels to you*
> *to hear Isabel's sadness about her mother and see her tears. Is she being a burden to us*
> *right now?" The response from the group was both warm and reassuring: They felt bet-*
> *ter for being able to comfort her. One husband said, "You are allowing your mother to*
> *be a mother to you."*

This feedback reflects the immediate experience in the group—the here-and-now—and carries far more power with it than discussions about a situation outside the room. It also allows the group to use their experience of one another to try out new ways of being and to receive feedback from people who care about them, but are not so close that the risk of trying something different is too high.

Some might consider such open discussion of serious problems nothing more than stirring up painful emotions with little potential for benefit. However, given the analogy we strive to create between interaction in the group and that in the real world of family and friends, the benefits outweigh the risks. Not surprisingly, patients report that their families are their primary source of emotional support (Primomo, Yates et al., 1990) and emotional concern (Liang, Dunn et al., 1990). The levels of distress are similar among patients and spouses (Kaye and Gracely, 1993; Kupst, 1993).

Husbands of cancer patients respond well to both information and emotional support (Northouse, 1989). Furthermore, we have found that certain types of family interaction at home predict how well the patients in the family will feel over time (Spiegel, Bloom et al. 1983). The more that family members supported one another, talked openly about problems, and reduced conflict, the less depressed were the patients over the ensuing years. In particular, expressiveness, a measure of shared and open problem solving, seems to be a reliable predictor of better family and patient coping with a variety of illnesses, ranging from Hodgkin's disease (Bloom, Fobair et al., 1991; Hannah, Gritz et al., 1992; Fobair, Hoppe et al., 1986) to breast cancer (Spiegel, Bloom et al., 1983) to schizophrenia (Spiegel and Wissler, 1983).

It pays to solve problems together rather than struggle with them separately. Our tendency is to hide what worries us the most from ourselves and from those closest to us. This creates isolation, impairs problem-solving, and seems to make patients sadder and more anxious. Conversely, the immediate sadness, fear, and tension created by discussing serious problems openly is more than offset by the reduction in subsequent unhappiness, among both cancer patients and their families. While it may be true that "misery loves company," it seems that company dispels misery.

> Sarah's daughter fought back the tears as she admitted to herself and the family group what she would lose when her mother died of breast cancer: "I've had lots of troubles in my life, lots of failures. Mom is the only person who always believes in me. I don't know what I will do without her." "Have you told your mom this?" was the question from several group members? "No," she replied, "I just feel so selfish—here I am worrying about myself, when she is dying." Laurie's mother gently confronted her: "You know, one day I said to my daughter, 'You are my best friend in the world.' She started to cry and I said: 'Didn't you know that?' 'Yes,' she replied, 'but it makes me feel so good to hear you say it.' Tell your Mom—it will make her feel important to you. That is not selfish at all."

Laurie's mother could play the part of Sarah to Sarah's daughter, reflecting how much it would mean to Sarah to hear her say plainly what her mother meant to her.

Clearly family members do not want to burden their ill loved ones with more problems than they need to absorb. This balance is not always easy to find, but groups can provide one way of evaluating what should be shared and what is too much. Groups can both stimulate interaction between family member and patient and provide an alternative place to unburden themselves. Just as cancer patients feel that it is fair to bring up anything in their group, since they both give and receive help, family members in the group setting are also relieved of the concern that they are burdening their ill family member with their concerns. Thus despite being among people they know less well than their families, they can have a lower threshold regarding what to discuss because the emotional consequences of telling too much are less than in their immediate family.

Coming to Terms with Dying.   Family groups become a means of coming to terms with and preparing for impending loss, often referred to by the members as a road map of what is to come. For many, the group is the first place where the emotional reality of the death of a loved one emerges. This occurs through confrontation with others who have suffered the loss or are closer to it. Many could not conceive of life without their loved ones. They observe over time others who were similarly unable to accept the possibility of this loss, and who have then gone through it. This makes the inconceivable real, which is painful, but it also demonstrates that people like themselves can get through it.

The therapists have multiple tasks in dealing with this difficult issue:

1. helping those most immediately affected by bad news, disease progression, or recent death to deal with those issues;
2. assessing the effect of such discussions on others in the group;
3. encouraging them to discuss their reactions to this threatening material; and
4. facilitating interaction between those immediately and more remotely affected.

"Tonight is the first time it seemed real to me that I could actually lose Shirley. I mean, I knew it would likely happen eventually, but it was just an idea. I am coming to see that it will happen, and it is shaking me," said Ed, a quiet engineer who spoke, like many men of his large stature, in an almost hushed baritone. "Who'll be my buddy?" he asked thoughtfully and sadly. Then he added, "I really don't have anyone else to talk

to about what I am struggling with. People expect me to just carry on. This group is a place where I come to feel better about feeling bad."

Often a therapist's inquiry about what seems to work best for others can elicit some useful strategies for dealing with difficult situations.

The therapist asked, "We've been discussing how hard it is to understand, let alone talk about, the possibility of losing your wife. Have you found a way to bring it up? What works?"

Carl talked about how his wife Nancy's proximity to death had led him to picture once or twice just what it would really mean to him if he knew that in days or weeks he might die. He told her of this experience: how upsetting it was to feel in this very personal way his own mortality. At the same time it helped him to better understand what she was going through, it also made him more aware that his own problems, pressures at work, and so on, were real too. While Nancy's problems were more immediate, his were just as real. At the same moment that he was more in touch with what she was going through, she could better feel what his difficulties were like. He said to the group that when he had told Nancy how close he had come to seeing what it was like for her, she reacted very warmly: "She gave me a massage. Then I said to her, 'I don't think I'd trade places, though.' Then she hit me. We had a good laugh about it."

There is an important element of anticipatory grief in these groups. A man whose wife is currently doing well faces another across the room whose disease is rapidly progressing. He can see that sooner or later he will be in the same position, but sees in front of him a man who earlier was as incredulous as he at the idea that he could lose his wife. This can be deeply upsetting. At the same time, however, he can see that someone like himself can get through such a trauma, can face life beyond the loss of his wife.

Group members can be encouraged to help one another through these difficult times with the help of active intervention by the leaders. Michael's story of the death of his wife, which we mentioned earlier, deeply affected others in the group.

"Michael, I know you lost Joanne just a little while ago. I'm sorry. Can you tell us what it was like for you?" Michael talked movingly about his final days with his wife: "During the last four days she was not really conscious. I had sent everybody else away—we were alone. I thought it would be better that way, but I never knew whether I was comforting or bothering her. I didn't want to leave her alone for fear that she'd suffer alone, but I didn't want to disturb her by being with her."

"What did you do?" the therapist asked.

"I just sat and read children's stories to her," he replied. "I didn't know whether she was annoyed or appreciated it. I never did get to say good-bye. I just couldn't do it."

The therapist responded, "I appreciate how hard this time has been for you, and how difficult it is to share it with us. We have a new member in the group—what is it like for you to hear this at your first meeting?"

The new member, Greg, responded, "It has been quite an experience for me—very moving. But it has shaken me somewhat, I have to admit."

"You know what?" said Michael. "The first meeting of the group that I was at somebody had just died and I heard the same thing. I want you to know that we had three wonderful years between that time and this. The three years after I had joined the group were better than the three years before."

Thus with encouragement from the therapist, the difficulty of both positions was acknowledged, and despite his intense grief, Michael was able to provide real comfort to Greg, which also helped him to develop a greater sense of mastery over his own loss. At the same time, he needed a place to grieve, and the group was providing it.

"Well, I guess I need a place to talk about Joanne. I feel like I'm not done talking about it and others seem to be pulling away. On the one hand, when I go to work, I want people to treat me as a person who is working and who can smile, and at the same time I need to talk about Joanne more. It is not just that I am facing the bigger picture of what I have lost, of the tragedy in it. I feel some sense of regret, wondering if I should have talked to her more about her fear of dying. Did she suffer it alone or did she really not feel it?"

The therapist said, "It sounds as though the turning point for you was when Joanne was no longer conscious, when she was lost to you as a companion." Michael pulled out of his pocket something he had received in the mail from a group celebrating the "heroes," the "survivors." He said, "You know, this really upset me when I read it because Joanne wasn't a survivor; we weren't survivors. You know this survivorship thing leaves out the people who die of the disease. If everyone were a survivor, we wouldn't be here." He then talked about how much this group meant to him, and how much Joanne had valued her group, although she hadn't gotten to tell them that directly. The therapist commented on how tenderly he had cared for Joanne during her illness, and the other men in the group told Michael how much the meeting had meant to them.

A recent death or worsening of disease in a group member's family is always a topic of primary importance. If it has occurred and the group is not discussing it, they should be. Take stock at the beginning of the group about who is absent and why, and whether there are any major changes or news to report. It is crucial that members facing an acute crisis not suffer in silence:

"Fred, I know that your problems at work are important, but Tom looks very upset and I wonder if we could take some time to find out what is upsetting him." Tom may then mention that his wife was told the adriamycin is no longer working, and "there is nothing else to do." "How did that leave you feeling?" would be a useful response.

The threat of loss and death is a primary concern, and the leaders must not collude in avoiding it.

Joe talked movingly about his grieving for Karen, who had died three months earlier. He mentioned a dream in which he was with her in an old Italian castle and suddenly he couldn't find her. She was gone and he was looking for her. When he saw her she was crying and coming toward him down a hill. The therapist asked him what happened next and he replied that he couldn't walk toward her. He said the dream was oddly comforting, although it was about Karen's death. He said he often deliberately kept weekends unscheduled so he could grieve more intensely for her. "Why was she crying?" asked the therapist. Joe said he had not thought of that before. Some of the comfort may have been his sense that she would have grieved for the loss of him just as he grieved her. He saw her tears, her fear of being separated from him, and her relief when she saw him in the dream. "You know," Joe said, "when I was late coming home from work Karen would say, 'I've made your funeral arrangements.'" He cried as he talked about the sweetness he recognized in her.

Discussion of dying and death is heavy going, but it builds closeness, and makes the group a unique place, where even the worst can be discussed. It is important that the therapists take every opportunity to raise questions about anticipatory grief and bereavement, and reinforce those who discuss it with empathic restatement of the issues raised.

Choosing Priorities.   One of the results of anticipatory grief is the ability to conceptualize and face the limited time that remains with loved ones. The importance of using that time well while attending to one's own life is emphasized. Members remind one another that they cannot be with their wives every minute, that they, too, are vulnerable and have their limits and needs.

Sam talked about how he and Annie had learned to negotiate, to express feelings rather than judgments. A retired gentleman, he disagreed gently with Michael, who said he felt he was not spending enough time with his wife. "On the contrary, I'm spending too much time with my wife. After retirement we have been together constantly and we find ourselves bickering as a way of maintaining our own domain. I find it important to spend some time by myself. When Annie asked me to visit her family in the East with her, I said, 'I'll stay for a week, but that's all I can take. I'm going to take a trip after that.' Annie said that was fine with her. He added that it made Annie feel good to be able to wish him some free time, although he always wondered if she would need him.

Such statements provide an opportunity for the therapist to inquire about others' response to the same problem: "How do others of you balance your own needs and those of your wives?" Such a statement summarizes but does not judge what has been said. It invites further discussion, acknowledging that it is legitimate for a husband to have some time to himself, even if his wife is very sick, but does not conclude that there is one "right way" to handle the situation.

Joe commented that he had come to realize how much he had been focused on work all of his life, for forty years being a scientist, and how much more there was to life: "It is as though I have suddenly opened my eyes—I can almost feel Karen applaud." He had gotten through much of his life and most of her death focusing on accomplishing things at work, but he was now becoming more interested in the personal and human dimension. The therapist pointed out that Sam's anticipation of his wife's death and Joe's loss of Karen had caused them to confront their own vulnerability and rethink their priorities in life.

John responded by talking about his constant irritation over little things: the computer not working properly, the harbor master giving them difficulties about their sailboat. The boat had been a great source of pleasure—something they had bought after Terry's diagnosis. "She looks so happy on that boat, and so relaxed. But I get so frustrated—with little things, with myself, with her." The therapist pursued this frustration: "What is it that sets you off?" He replied that it was the constraints placed on them by her illness, coupled with her working very hard, and his limited income. The little things were just triggers for the big ones.

The threat posed by the illness often stimulates husbands and children to reevaluate their priorities. Some men cut back to part-time jobs, and others undertake new recreational activities or travel. The therapist's task is then to acknowledge the tension that can lead to reevaluation: "If you can't do as much, how do you decide what has to go?" is an example of such a question. Also, as much as possible, the therapist is charged with broadening the applicability of the issue, inquiring of other group members whether they have had similar experiences or problems. Group therapy is not just a series of individual therapy sessions. Each problem expressed is an opportunity for deepening the sense of commonality, broadening the repertoire of responses, and helping members feel understood and accepted even if there is no complete agreement about the right thing to do.

Revising Family Relationships.   Understandably, a good deal of time is spent discussing family relationships, often from the point of view of exchanging ideas about what works. This kind of information swapping is useful in that it acknowledges common problems, gives members a sense of competence in being able to offer suggestions to others, and broadens their repertoire of responses.

(a) Role Flexibility. "Life may be better after cancer, but it will never be the same," said one cancer patient. While there is often a desperate effort to maintain a semblance of normalcy and sameness after cancer has been diagnosed, it is rarely possible. Cancer treatment and the progression of the disease, if it occurs, will inevitably place constraints on the abilities of the ill family member. She cannot do what she used to do, so others must fill in. However, the ill family member may be able (and want) to take on some other tasks in return.

Role flexibility involves reexamining who does what in the family and reassigning roles based on the changing medical circumstances. The husband may have to learn to cook and clean, while the wife can take over paying the bills. These changes are often difficult, because they require acknowledging the impact of the disease, a kind of grief work that involves admitting and bearing losses. At the same time, doing so acknowledges that all members of the family have needs and responsibilities, even though they may have to be shuffled because of the impact of the disease.

Some flexibility is also needed in the way men and women typically respond to stress. Men frequently express the desire to respond to a problem by fixing it. The model is the broken car: Find the defective part and replace it, then everything will be fine. However, a woman with serious illness may not feel fixable. She may be unhappy about her illness and what it means, and want someone to sympathize with her. Her husband's however well-intended desire to fix the problem is often experienced by her as a desire to avoid it.

This situation has been likened to one in which a couple has an electric blanket with dual controls that have been crossed. She is cold so she turns up the temperature. He starts to feel too hot, so he turns his down. She feels even colder, and turns hers up more, and so on. Conversely, a man ill with prostate cancer may well feel frustrated or even humiliated by sympathy from his wife because he wants to fix the problem. Difficulties in sexual performance may form a template for this frustration—he does not want to be understood, which can make him feel even weaker because he wants the problem to go away. It can help if a wife comes to understand that sympathy which might make her feel better could make her husband feel worse. Instead she might offer comfort by acknowledging the things he does or still can do that make her feel fulfilled in various ways, sexually and otherwise.

Bridging the gap between the desire to fix rather than to understand and accept a problem is illustrated in the following group interaction:

> *The therapist asked, "So what does it feel like when your wife seems so unhappy?" John responded, "I just want to do something to make her feel better. But every time I try something, she just seems more depressed or she gets angry at me. One evening Terry was just so frustrated. I'd never seen her like that before. Normally she is a ball of energy. But she was feeling so weak and tired and sick that she couldn't even get up out of the chair. I just didn't know what to do anymore, so I just gave up and gave her a hug and we both cried. It turned out that was the right thing to do. Just when I thought I had blown it."*

Getting the men in this group to take a look at their own helplessness allowed them to see that their tendency to fix things is a response to this unbearable sense of helplessness, rather than "the only sensible thing to do." They then found that just sharing the frustration with their wives was a better response than trying to push it aside. They thus used their own array of experiences to broaden their modes of responding to their wives' distress.

(b) Open Communication. Needs will not be met until they are recognized. Spouses and other family members are often in a savior mode, feeling they should sacrifice all for their loved one who is ill, and showing little interest in looking after their own needs and wishes. There are times when such inequality in the give-and-take of a family is necessary and helpful.

However, over the long haul it wears thin. Frustrations build, tempers flare, and there are often blow-ups over apparently inconsequential matters.

In the same family group Michael, the husband of a woman with advanced breast cancer, both hardworking professionals, recounted their "taco fight." His wife, Joanne, had built a prominent career, and found herself increasingly frustrated by the limitations her disease imposed. She had been so determined to pursue her work that she went on a business trip to Australia, despite metastatic disease. During the trip she fell in a darkened theater, breaking her leg (the fall was accidental, but the fracture was due in part to metastases to the bones in her legs).

Some months later after she had recovered, she was preparing dinner with a kind of grim determination ("At least I can do this"). She realized as she was about to serve the dinner that she had forgotten the lettuce. Her husband and son both immediately volunteered to go out and get some. Beyond frustration with her inability to do even something so simple as prepare a dinner, she screamed: "What is the matter with you? Can't you eat tacos without lettuce?" They were stunned, thinking they had just been trying to be helpful. On reflection in the group, the husband realized that had he said, "We don't need lettuce," she probably would have yelled: "Won't one of you even go to the store and get some lettuce? Why won't anyone help?" He realized that his wife, a highly competent woman, was struggling with the cruel limitations that the illness placed upon her.

Ed, another man in the group, said, "You know, I keep trying to be helpful and it doesn't work. There are times when my wife just gets mad and everything I try is wrong. She bites my head off for no reason. Finally one day I just started to cry and said, 'Honey, I don't know what to do to help you.' We hugged each other and she cried and we felt much better. "What did Ed do that was so helpful?" inquired the therapist. "He stopped trying to be helpful," mused Mark. "I am always trying to be useful, helpful." The therapist said, "And all that does for your wife is highlight her feelings of incompetence. Ed got a lot farther when he admitted that he felt every bit as incompetent to deal with the situation as his wife did." Michael said, "As a man, I always just want to fix things, make them better. But that's not what my wife wants. She wants support: words, not deeds."

Thus, the men came to be more aware of and comfortable admitting that they did not know what to do, and that acting as though they did only made matters worse. They could try admitting their own helplessness and becoming more aware of it. They felt freer to do this because they were not immediately confronted with their wives' frustrations, but rather with other men who were in the same boat.

However, a more powerful means of deepening members' understanding of what is going on in their families is the use of the process as information about what may need improvement at home. "How can we help you?" is often a useful question from a group leader to a troubled member.

George's wife was rapidly declining, and he said he was becoming more depressed as he watched this. Nonetheless, he showed very little emotion. "This is a very difficult situation for you," said the therapist, "but I am not clear what I can do to help you with it." "Nothing," responded George. "My wife is dying. What can you do?" "We can try to help you cope with it," responded another man in the group. "Sometimes when I feel overwhelmed, I just need a hug. I keep trying to fix things and then it gets to be one too many and I can't take it. I just want a hug," said another. George began to see that in his despair he was not letting us help him, and how he could get more of the support he needed by being more aware of and open about his own needs and emotions.

The co-therapists are in a kind of family relationship as well, and group members will watch their interaction closely. They can model the kind of respectful difference of opinion that facilitates open communication in families: "I think I know what David had in mind when he said that, but I was more concerned that we changed the course of the discussion before you got to say what you wanted to. Was there more you intended to tell us?" This kind of interaction can be a model for the group in ways to negotiate differences within families. This kind of interaction among therapists also models the idea that effective collaboration and mutual help do not require complete agreement. The therapists can work together without having the same perspective on every issue. This provides a model for respectful differences in families: spouses and patients do inevitably have different points of view. They need not agree on everything to effectively help each other.

Revising Doctor-Patient and Doctor-Family Relationships. The sense of helplessness engendered by the illness is often reflected by frustration about doctor-patient interactions. The therapist will inevitably experience transference of feelings from physicians, usually in the form of challenges regarding the purpose and direction of the group.

Group members sometimes wonder aloud what the exact purpose of the group is, and why the leader is not clearer about it. It is important that the leader be open and responsive to such challenges, rather than defensive. Group leaders are not there to make the members comfortable. Indeed, often their questions stir discomfort, and there can be no promises of magical cure. They are asking something very difficult of group members: to discuss inner feelings of dread, to revise life priorities, and to restructure family relationships. At least they can be open to challenges: "I see that the group process does not seem clear to you. Is that true for others in the group?" This legitimates the question, and invites confirmation or disagreement from other members.

After hearing the concerns, the leader can provide an answer: "We hope that the group will help you clarify what your needs, feelings, and concerns are so that you can learn to get more of what you need in your family, from your medical consultations, and elsewhere in your life."

Thus, through these interactions with the therapists, group members can try out what it would be like to challenge their doctors. Such challenges are best responded to with open acknowledgment and exploration, rather than avoidance or dismissal. This models effective and assertive interaction with physicians, showing that professionals can and should tolerate challenges to their authority and knowledge. Use such interactions as an occasion to reinforce the group members' risk taking. For instance, the following response by the therapist gives the members permission to state their real concerns: "I know it is not easy to raise such uncomfortable questions about the direction of the group with me. I appreciate your doing it. Let's explore what your concerns are so that I can respond to them."

It is also important that the boundary between group therapy and individual medical care be meticulously respected. Questions about individual prognosis or treatment must be deflected back to the treating physician: "I think that is a very important question, but one that only your doctor can answer. I suggest that you take it up with him/her." The focus is on clarifying questions rather than providing answers. The therapist can underscore that the family has the right to know answers, and encourage husbands to attend physician visits with their wives.

The group process can also be used to model clarification of communication with physicians. Families and patients often confuse wanting more information from doctors with wanting better news. For instance, "John, I hear you telling us that you can't get straight answers from your doctors about your wife's prognosis. But what I hear also is that when doctors have told you bad news about the future, you challenge them. Could you try out with us what your question to the doctor might be?" Often a family member's understandable ambivalence about hearing the truth may cloud communication with physicians: They want the truth but they want it to be good news. Helping them to sort through these conflicting desires may allow them to clarify questions and allow them to better accept the answers. At the same time, there may be situations in which the family and patient are quite clear, and the doctors are just plain unwilling to provide needed information.

Family members often experience a special sense of helplessness in their interactions with doctors: They depend upon a relative stranger for the life of a person who is precious to them. In addition to the usual authority conferred by professional status, family members often sense that they are in danger of alienating much-needed help if they challenge doctors at all. This can lead them to avoid discussing difficult issues, and at the same time resent the inevitable lack of responsiveness to these issues. Family groups can provide a forum for trying out different means of raising concerns, clarifying information, and participating appropriately in decision making.

GROUPS FOR
OTHER ILLNESSES

The supportive-expressive group therapy model is relevant to all kinds of chronic, debilitating, and life-threatening illnesses. Receiving a diagnosis of any serious illness will have many psychosocial consequences similar to those we have discussed. Being diagnosed with a serious illness will reinforce some or all of the existential concerns that we have outlined—the sense of isolation, a radically altered identity, a need to reorder priorities or to redefine oneself, and, with some illnesses, a fear of death. In addition, there is often an effect on the family and social relationships.

While there may be many similarities, it is also important to acknowledge the differences between various illnesses. For example, we noted the similarities and differences between living with primary breast cancer and living with metastatic disease. Recognizing the unique issues that arise for different patients is crucial for the success of any group. In this section, we draw on our experience with other serious illnesses to illustrate some of the differences that can emerge.

HIV INFECTION

Working with individuals who are infected with the human immunodeficiency virus (HIV), some of whom may have developed acquired immuno-

deficiency syndrome (AIDS), presents a host of issues for the group therapist to bear in mind (Kelly, Murphy et al., 1993). While it is not possible to do
this topic justice, we will present some of our observations and experiences
in working with HIV-infected individuals.

Dealing with Diverse Populations.   We have found that the most effective HIV
groups are those groups where members share similar backgrounds (which
usually pertains to how they got infected) and are of the same gender. Certainly this is not absolutely imperative but it is similar to our experiences in
working with primary and metastatic breast cancer patients, where these
women shared many issues but also differed in important ways. The issues
that HIV patients struggle with have many similarities and differences; the
differences are important because they often go to the core of who these people are and what they struggle with.

For instance, most (but certainly not all) men who are infected with HIV
are gay. There is a culture and lifestyle that gay men identify with that sets
them apart from other infected individuals. We led one HIV group for men
and, as it turned out, all were gay except for Charlie. Not only was Charlie
set apart because he was heterosexual, he was also a former IV drug user.
Thus, the culture that Charlie came from was different on several accounts.
Charlie was an affable guy, who was perhaps more disclosing and talkative
than he should be.

> *During the first session, Charlie revealed that he was straight and that he had been in-
> fected through his drug use. Although the other members seemed to genuinely like
> Charlie and tried to relate to him, it was clear that he was too different from them. If he
> had only differed on one account, perhaps this group would have worked for him. How-
> ever, as the weeks passed and as Charlie revealed more and more about himself and his
> struggles, Charlie also seemed to become increasingly more distressed by the group and
> in response the other group members became increasingly more distant. Eventually,
> Charlie decided that the group was not for him. Although this was an unfortunate out-
> come for everyone concerned, there was also a positive side to this development. Because
> the group was now solely comprised of gay men, they could spend more time talking
> about issues that pertained to being both gay and infected.*

If it is at all possible, we recommend having separate groups for men and
women, and separate groups for people who have been infected through IV

drug use, unsafe sex, or prostitution. There is already so much stigma attached to having HIV that creating a group environment that facilitates understanding and acceptance is of the utmost importance.

For groups composed of individuals who have become infected through IV drug use, there are often other compounding factors. For some, they might still struggle with their addiction. We have had individuals in our groups who were not clean and sober but who nevertheless wanted to experience the benefits of a support group. Surprisingly, some of these individuals have been some of our most valuable and valued members. Participation in a group should be restricted, however, to those who are not under the influence of drugs or alcohol. This is important for both the member who uses but also for those who are clean and sober. For those members who are clean and sober an intoxicated member in the group can be distressing. Seeing someone under the influence is often distressing because it can activate others' desires to use drugs and alcohol. For the member who is intoxicated, on the other hand, the benefits or contributions that can be made to the group are limited by their impaired functioning.

Another compounding factor in groups of individuals infected through IV drug use is that many of them come from chaotic backgrounds, including but not limited to poverty. This lack of resources may restrict their ability to attend the group regularly or may present difficulties in securing transportation to the group. These are obstacles that, while not insurmountable, can present considerable challenges to conducting effective groups. For this population, we recommend holding your group in a place that is convenient and familiar to the members.

In our groups for women, we discovered that the community of HIV-infected women was a relatively small one and that consequently many of these women knew each other outside of group. This raised special concerns regarding confidentiality, and careful discussions were required to be sure that everyone felt they could trust that the content of their group discussions was confidential.

Illness-Related Issues. The field of HIV treatment is rapidly changing. For example, we wrote a grant proposal to examine the benefits for HIV-positive patients of participating in our support groups with the expectation that we would help patients deal with the inevitability of dying from AIDS. By the time we got the grant and started the study, highly active anti-retroval therapy (HAART) was introduced, and now the one question that was upper-most in the minds of HIV-infected individuals was not "How do I prepare for dying?" but rather "How do I now prepare for living?"

As the years have passed the complexities of following a HAART regi-men and the uncertainty about who will benefit and for how long has be-come more apparent. Being infected with HIV is no longer an automatic death sentence. Instead, the patient might be faced with managing a chronic disease or, alternatively, facing a slow and steady march toward death.

There are multiple physical issues with which HIV-infected patients must contend: the constant risk of opportunistic infections; the battle with fatigue, anemia, and wasting; the ongoing concern with viral load and T cell count; and the demands of treatment adherence, which requires that medications be taken several times a day, some with food, some without food, and some with horrible side effects.

Existential Issues.   HIV infects more than the body; it infects the entire per-son. HIV immediately raises the specter of death and all the concerns that surround death and the dying process. For HIV patients, concern about dy-ing is often compounded by the fact that their infection may have made them outcasts from their support system. Thus, there may be a realistic fear of dying alone, which only compounds feelings of isolation. Because of the stigma of being infected, patients are naturally reluctant to tell others about their illness, further adding to their isolation.

Finding meaning with an illness such as this can be a real challenge. Re-ordering priorities is inevitable as the patient is required to adjust to a changed body and, ultimately, to a changed world including relationships, lifestyle, and a sense of the future.

Damaged Social Support System.   HIV infection is perhaps the most devastat-ing illness in terms of altering and frequently destroying relationships. Worse still, it is often the most important relationships that are destroyed, such as those with parents, siblings, and lovers. The effects of losing or dam-aging these relationships are very painful and consequently elicit strong emotion, which places the support group in an especially vital role. Helping patients mourn the loss of important relationships and to nurture damaged relationships is an important goal, as is building new and supportive relationships within the group. Group members have a special role to play in helping to replace what has been lost.

Multiple Sclerosis

Characteristics of the Illness.   Multiple sclerosis (MS) typically affects adults between the ages of twenty and fifty. Little is known about what causes the disease or who is more likely to get it. It is not considered a fatal disease, although a small percentage of people do die from it; it is instead a disease that is characterized by remissions and exacerbations when the disease flares up.

Some people have a mild form of MS and others a more severe form. Approximately one-quarter to one-third will end up in a wheelchair. Symptoms include fatigue (which is sometimes overwhelming), loss of coordination, muscle weakness and spasms, slurred speech, numbness, visual difficulties, and cognitive impairment. Acute but less frequent symptoms include paralysis, bowel and bladder dysfunction, muscle cramps, and sexual dysfunction.

Psychological Issues.   Psychologically, one of the most difficult aspects of MS is its unpredictability. Patients will complain that they never know what state their body will be in when they wake up in the morning. Because of its unpredictability, some patients will simply use denial and on those days when their bodies aren't how they should be, they will simply ignore it and proceed as though nothing were wrong.

> One of our group members, Doug, was notorious for this, so much so that it became a standing joke. Eventually, both the group leaders and members would use humor to help him recognize the foolhardiness of his behavior. For instance, he would routinely ignore what his body was telling him and then spend the day carrying out a physically taxing and often precarious job that would frequently put him in physically vulnerable situations. With the ongoing support of the group, he got better and better at recognizing when he was doing this and eventually was able to gain control over this tendency. At the same time he also realized that this expressed his struggle to avoid the reality of his illness.

Related to the unpredictability of MS is uncertainty about what the course of the disease will be. In some the course is worse than in others, and so, with every exacerbation there is anxiety about the disease's course. Hearing the experiences of other group members and how they handled their exacerbations is often very helpful during this time.

Depression is common among MS patients. It can be a reaction to having the disease but can also be caused by it. Thus, it is important to encourage depressed patients to seek a psychiatric medication evaluation. The support of the group is also important during this time. Learning how others have coped with the debilitating effects of the illness and also having a place to talk about their concerns are vitally important.

Similar to other serious illnesses, MS will activate existential concerns. Coming to terms with a changed identity is a central challenge for the MS patient. So too are issues pertaining to meaning and freedom. However remote, the threat of death is likely to stimulate death anxiety in some patients.

LUPUS

Characteristics of the Illness. Systemic lupus erythematosus (SLE) is a lifelong, potentially fatal, autoimmune disease. Similar to MS, it is characterized by unpredictable exacerbations and remissions. It is also similar to HIV infection in that it can involve multiple organs, may be life-threatening, and can require careful monitoring. Lupus causes inflammation of various parts of the body, including the skin, joints, blood, kidneys, lungs, heart, nervous system, and/or other body organs or systems. Common symptoms include achy joints, fever, prolonged or extreme fatigue, arthritis, skin rashes, and anemia. The kidneys can be involved. There can be pain upon breathing, hair loss, and sun or light sensitivity.

Psychological Issues. The psychological issues characteristic of MS are similar to the issues experienced by lupus patients. The patient must learn to cope with the unpredictability and uncertainty of the disease and also the potential threat of death.

Another characteristic that cuts across these issues and that is shared by these illnesses is a lack of control.

> *Doreen told the group that she had learned the results of her MRI and it showed that the lupus was affecting her brain and that there was little that they could do about it since drugs can't get through the blood/brain barrier. The therapist responded, "Gee, that's*

really—" with Doreen finishing her sentence: "—serious." Then Doreen said, "So I was really down for a few days but now I've come to terms. . . . Like you said, I have to accept it. I can't do so much. Because my memory is really bad. It's really hard." This clearly was devastating news. Perhaps that was why she so glibly went on to say that she just needed to accept it. Certainly, there was more beneath the surface that needed examination. At this point the therapist simply ignored her statements about how she would cope and said, "Doreen, can you say a little more about what it was like to hear that the lupus has affected your brain?" This enabled Doreen to talk about the emotional devastation she was feeling.

Concerns regarding unpredictability can emerge in many ways.

Michelle told the group that for the first time she was really thinking about lupus and how unpredictable it is. She stated that she worried about what else could happen and that she wanted to get a copy of her medical records to help her predict what might happen. This was a clear statement of Michelle's desire to have some control over her disease. There was a pause and then Mary stated that she was concerned that she caused her own problems by thinking about them. This appeared to another way of expressing a desire for control. If thinking was a way of causing problems, then this suggested that she had a means to control them.

As in the other illnesses we have discussed, lupus raises existential concerns pertaining to death, isolation, meaning, and freedom. By extrapolation, we hope it is evident that existential concerns are activated by any chronic, debilitating, or potentially life-threatening disease.

CONCLUSION

There is much that is family-like about groups. Members care about one another and become close, but also need to have their own independence of thought and action. They can try out means of interacting with one another for later use in their families. They can also enact roles in the group complementary to those at home: a mother talking to a daughter, one spouse reflecting on the stress borne by another. At times, members can be more open and honest within the group than at home because they are less closely involved. The therapist's role is to push for open exploration of affect, seek common themes, encourage the development of new ways of coping, and provide support.

The commonality of experience within such groups allows for exploration of personal and stressful problems. The fact that group members are like family but yet not family provides an environment for testing out thoughts, feelings, and coping strategies. The atmosphere of openness and direct confrontation with serious problems created in the group can become a model for a similar working through of problems in the family.

Supportive-expressive group therapy is applicable to all types of serious illnesses. In this chapter we briefly described three different illnesses in order to demonstrate both similarities and differences. It was not our intention to be exhaustive regarding the relevance of supportive-expressive group therapy to other illnesses nor did we attempt to provide a thorough discussion of the issues that arise in each of these diseases; we hope that this discussion provided sufficient examples to illustrate the range of both common and unique issues that can arise.

CHAPTER 10

Group Problems

It is the rare group that will be problem-free. In fact, if you think that you have one of those groups, you might ask yourself "Is there something I am not seeing?" Every group will have its rough spots, some worse than others. There might be a challenging member, an upsetting event, a difficult group process, or a group that is so "nice" that they avoid the tough issues. In this chapter we discuss some of the different types of problems that you may encounter. We hope that these illustrative examples will provide you with the tools you need to address any problem that may arise.

CONFRONTATIONS
AMONG GROUP MEMBERS

Bob was the newest member of an established group for HIV positive gay men. He was a somewhat insecure, complex, and thoughtful young man. He had been diagnosed a few months before and was feeling isolated and in need of a new support system. From the moment he entered the group, it was clear that this was a sensitive young man who was fairly easily put on the defensive. Over time we learned that this came out of a history of rejection in his family. Bob and Jonathon never quite hit it off. Their viewpoints were often at odds and each had a stubborn side to him that prevented a real meeting of the minds.

Peter, on the other hand, was "Mr. Diplomacy." He always found a way to see everyone's point of view and consequently was genuinely liked by everyone. Jonathon and Peter had become fast friends, and it was clear that they spent a lot of time together outside of the group.

Over the weeks, the tension between Bob and Jonathon mounted. The therapists worked hard to help them talk about the issues between them but inevitably one of them would say something that the other found offensive. One day, it finally came to a head. At the end of his rope, Jonathon said, "I don't think I can be in this group any longer. This is not a support group if all I get is criticism from Bob. I've had it. I'm leaving." Jonathon stood up and prepared to leave. The group leaders urged Jonathon to stay so that they could work it out. Jonathon refused and left.

This presented a dilemma for the group leaders. What should they do? The group leaders looked at each other and one said to the other, "I think one of us should go and catch Jonathon and talk to him. What do you think?" "I agree," said the co-leader; "I'll go." The unstated goal of the leaders was to try to get beneath Jonathon's anger and access his hurt feelings and then to encourage him to return to the group and to speak about why he was feeling hurt. At the same time, the group leader who remained behind adopted the same strategy with Bob.

As it turned out, what lay beneath the surface for Bob were feelings of envy about Jonathon and Peter's relationship outside of group. These feelings were so tender that Bob had been unable to state them and thus they were expressed through his criticism of Jonathon. Jonathon, on the other hand, felt deeply hurt by what he described as Bob's constant jabs. Like Bob, Jonathon also came from a family that had rejected him. Thus, both Bob and Jonathon were replaying old family dynamics such that intense feelings were being elicited. Understanding what the group dynamic was triggering in each of them was crucial for helping them reach a level of understanding and acceptance.

Fortunately, confrontations such as these are rare in supportive-expressive groups, the reason being that the focus of these groups is on providing support to one another. This is in contrast to psychotherapy groups where the focus is on personality change. In psychotherapy groups it is not unusual for conflict to occur and is considered grist for the mill. In support groups conflict is contrary to the group culture and works against the goals of the group as this example so clearly illustrated.

Occasionally, however, confrontations do occur. In such situations the task of the leader is to function as a mediator and to help facilitate caring and supportive communication. Since the purpose of the group is to explore the impact the illness has had on each of the members and to provide support to one another, it is likely that the conflict is in some way related to these concerns. The leader should ask herself or himself, as well as the members concerned, "In what way is this conflict tied to the group process?" It may be, as we saw in this example, that someone is feeling left out and hurt feelings are coming out as anger. Or, it may be that one member is frustrated because the other member is thwarting the group process. The accused member may be doing so because of intense anxiety about his or her illness. Whatever the conflict may be, the goal of the leader is to help the members arrive at an understanding about the deeper meaning to the conflict. If the group has maintained its focus on the illness, then it is highly likely that conflict revolves around that focus as well.

SCAPEGOATING

Let us return to the case of Melanie, whose cancer metastasized while she was a member of an early-stage breast cancer group.

During the meeting when Melanie made her grim announcement and asked her question about whether the group members would still welcome her, it was important to her that she receive a response from everyone. As the members responded, there was a strong message of support that was being given to Melanie, until they heard from Loretta.

From the very first group meeting, it had been clear that Loretta was a little different from the others. She spoke in a monotone voice, expressed little affect, and on several occasions referred to having been hospitalized for psychiatric problems. She began in her usual monotone: "I was in another support group once." This response was enough to let the other group members know that they weren't going to like what they were about to hear. The nonverbal cues spoke volumes. The woman beside her suddenly got up and moved her chair as far away from Loretta as she could. Other members began to stare at the floor or to look straight ahead. Another woman glanced anxiously back and forth between Loretta and Melanie. Melanie looked a little dazed. The point of Loretta's story was that she had been in a group that had faced a similar situation and they too invited the woman to stay but the woman eventually died.

The group sat in stunned silence after Loretta's story, with some glaring openly at Loretta. "I don't get what you are saying, Loretta," one member said in angry confrontation. "Neither do I," said another, equally angry. It was clear that there were some difficult feelings in the room, feelings that were there prior to Loretta's ill-fated attempt at support, and that Loretta had just made herself an easy target. The group leader said, "Loretta, it seems that there might be a few things that you are trying to tell us with your story. I wonder if you could start with the most important point first. What is the message you are trying to convey with this story? Do you want Melanie to stay in our group?" "Yes, I do. Very much," she replied. "Is it hard for you to tell her that di-

rectly?" the therapist probed. "I've never been very good at being direct," Loretta explained. "I really didn't mean anything bad by my story. I just wanted to let everyone know what happened."

The other facilitator observing the interchange between Loretta and the co-leader as well as the reactions of the other group members said, "You know, I'm wondering about something. Your story, Loretta, seems to have stirred up some difficult feelings in the group. But, I'm wondering if those difficult feelings are really about you and the fact that you told this story. Perhaps it's because you've just told us a story that we all know might be the story of our group. You just described something that secretly everyone one of us is fearing might happen in here." This interpretation named the elephant in the room that Loretta had unwittingly pointed to. By identifying the real issue, the group members, including Melanie, were able to talk about these dark fears.

Scapegoating is a way of deflecting attention away from an uncomfortable issue, in this case the fear that Melanie would die, and displacing the negative affect that issue evokes onto someone else. If scapegoating occurs in supportive-expressive groups, it should be concluded that the group is engaged in a major attempt to avoid dealing with some anxiety-provoking topic and that this topic has to do with the illness. The person who is scapegoated may represent the topic in some way. On the other hand, the scapegoated woman may simply be the easiest target. Whatever the situation, scapegoating is destructive and the leaders must protect the person who is scapegoated and help the group recognize the real issue they are avoiding. If the scapegoating is not dealt with and eliminated, it will undermine the integrity of the group, and all members, not just the woman being scapegoated, will suffer. On the other hand, identifying the source of the problem is likely to facilitate discussions about core issues.

THE MONOPOLIZER

A common problem in groups is the monopolizing patient. This is someone who finds it very difficult to be quiet in the group, jumps to speak at every opportunity, and has a hard time giving up the floor. Not only do these patients tend to monopolize the conversation and make it difficult for others to speak, but they typically do not speak about things of real substance or importance. The main reason for the constant verbiage is anxiety (Yalom, 1995). The monopolizer is anxious if silent and thus talks to quell it. The effect that the monopolizing patient has on the group is to instill frustration and create distance between the monopolizer and others.

It is important that therapists intervene early on in the evolution of the group so as to circumvent the development of such a problem. The problem is twofold: One is to help the monopolizer; the other is to protect the group. As Yalom (1995) describes it, the aim is not to get the monopolizer to speak less, but to have her speak more.

Eventually, the therapist will have to interrupt the monopolizer and help her to speak from a more meaningful place. In order to do this, the leaders will need to closely attend to what the patient says and also its context. You may notice that she tends to claim the floor immediately after someone has said something distressing. In such a case, an appropriate intervention would be to interrupt her and to ask how she felt about what she had just heard.

If it is difficult for the patient to access his or her immediate experience, it may be necessary to follow the question with an interpretive statement such as "I'm wondering if you felt a need to change the topic to something that is not so upsetting." Certainly, these kinds of interventions have to be done sensitively and respectfully. The goal of the group is not personality change. Consequently, the strategy is to try to work with the personalities as they are and, at the same time, to facilitate each member in dealing with the many issues that have arisen for her because of the cancer.

Another strategy in dealing with a monopolizing patient is to elicit reactions from the rest of the group. Again, this must be done sensitively. The strategy is to ask for reactions in a way that will facilitate the expression of supportive statements. The person who is monopolizing needs to feel that the rest of the group wants to hear about her concerns, feelings, and anxieties.

Whenever the monopolizer reveals thoughts and feelings of any importance, this presents a perfect opportunity to elicit reactions from the group. This approach will help the patient feel heard and valued as a person and will encourage her to communicate at a more meaningful level.

THE SILENT MEMBER

On the surface, silent patients can seem to pose much less of a problem than monopolizers. In some respects, however, they can prove to be even more difficult. One of the reasons is that silence can be an expression of any number of things. The silence may be due to fears about performance, feeling intimidated, feelings of superiority, fears about opening up the dam within, or discomfort in self-revelation.

The goal with silent patients is to help them break through their silence. For some, being called upon to speak can be distressing. Consequently, it is important to be careful in how you invite participation. In the early stages of the group, an open question about group reactions can be asked in such a way that it does not single out particular individuals. If your silent members do not respond, they can be turned to directly. If someone remains relatively silent for the first two or three groups, it will be necessary to address her directly. The therapist can comment on the silence and inquire about her impressions of the group. The hope is that this will enable the patient to break the ice and begin to participate. In all likelihood, even if this does work, the leaders will need to continue supporting the patient as she is drawn out. If over the course of time these approaches fail, the leaders may choose to address the question more directly in the group. Alternatively, the leaders may want to speak with the patient on an individual basis in an effort to understand the problem.

As in the case of the monopolizing patient, the group can be drawn on to support the silent member. They can be asked for their reactions to the silence. This question should be asked in the context of the leaders stating their concern for the patient. The aim is to create as supportive and caring an environment for the silent member as possible. The more the other members can be utilized to do this, the more effective it will be.

Although it is important to be careful about talking about people when they are absent, there are times when it can be helpful. In a situation in which there is a silent member and efforts have been made to draw the member into the group discussion, it might be helpful to talk about this issue in the member's absence. However, we advise that this discussion be initiated by the group members and not the group leaders. We see no good reason for the group leaders to initiate the discussion, unless there are veiled references to the issue. However, technically speaking, veiled references to the issue are just another way of group members bringing up the issue. Group members might want to bring up the issue because they have felt uncomfortable with addressing their concerns in the silent member's presence. For this reason it is helpful to facilitate a discussion of the members' concerns. The focus should be on helping the members examine why they have had difficulty raising the issue directly with the silent member. The general rule of thumb is to approach these discussions with the assumption that anything stated in the member's absence will be reported to the member upon her return. It is not necessary that this be done in all cases, such as when members inquire about members who are ill or if they pass along information about absent members. However, when there are important discussions about a member in her absence, it is crucial that the gist of these discussions be told to the absent member. Otherwise, you run the risk of creating a dysfunctional group environment where secrets are kept from one or more members. Thus, the group needs to be reminded that this issue must be brought up again when the silent member returns. The group may need help in planning a comfortable way to broach the topic.

Just because a patient is silent does not mean that she has not benefited from the group. Although silent, she may be listening intently and be deeply engaged in the group process. The silent member can still experience the support of the group and feel the acceptance of its members. Even so, the group leaders should not forget about this member, but continue in their efforts to engage her in the group discussions.

THE "SPECIAL" MEMBER

The "special" patient feels set apart, different from the rest of the group, and uses the differences that she sees as a way to detach from the group. In this way the patient is able to disengage emotionally from difficult topics.

Muriel is a clinical psychologist with cancer. She decided to join a support group because as a mental health professional she knew that support groups were supposed to be helpful. Although she intended to participate, it seemed that the only role she was willing to play in the group was as a psychologist. Muriel sat back and listened, occasionally offering her observations and sometimes offering advice. Rarely did she speak about herself.

One meeting, another group member had spent a good deal of the session describing the turmoil she was in because of her cancer and the quality of her intimate relationship. Muriel had been listening quietly and when she finally spoke up she began by saying, "As I've been sitting here, listening with my third ear . . ." and then went on to give her observations.

"Listening with my third ear" was an obvious reference to her listening as a therapist listens. The therapists both caught the reference and decided it was time to address the issue of her not participating as a group member.

The therapist commented, "Muriel, I was struck by your remark that you were 'listening with your third ear,' suggesting that you were not listening as a group member but as a therapist. Is this how you experience yourself in the group—as another therapist rather than a group member? I know it is how I experience you." "I don't think so," she said. "I also know I can't help what I know." This attempt to deny and rebuff the intervention of the group leader was intended to shut down this line of inquiry.

The co-leader decided to step in and try another tactic. "Given that you do know so much about human nature and therapy, I wonder if it might feel to you that there isn't very much that the group can offer you?" she asked.

This was an attempt on the part of the therapist to describe Muriel's inner experience. By being empathic, Muriel might be better able to talk about what was going on internally.

Muriel answered tentatively, "Well, maybe. Although I do find it interesting to hear what other people have to say and to hear about their experiences." "By just listening though, I imagine that ends up leaving you alone with your pain. I can't help but wonder how the group can help you if you don't tell us about yourself," the therapist replied.

In this intervention the therapist first gives an empathic statement about Muriel being left alone with her pain. Feeling this empathic connection with the group leader made her less defensive and therefore more open to the next question:

"How can we help you if you don't tell us about yourself?" This resulted in Muriel finally opening herself up to the group.

"Well, you're probably right. I was hoping that I could use this group but I find myself sitting back and getting very analytical. I'm not sure why. Maybe it's just easier," Muriel stated. "Easier than what?" the other therapist inquired. Muriel responded, "When I first came to group I found it upsetting to hear about people's recurrences. I don't want to get sad. I just want to put the cancer out of my mind. It seems I only have feelings about the cancer when I come here. I guess listening as a therapist allows me to get some distance on it all."

Muriel had just described the crux of the problem and, in so doing, had revealed her main struggle. This breakthrough was important for both her and the group. She had finally become a member of the group.

There are many ways in which a patient can decide to see herself as special and set apart from the group. The patient might compare her disease to those of the other patients and conclude that hers is not as serious. Therefore, many of the issues that the group is concerned with are not relevant to her situation. The patient might use religion: "God is my healer and source of support, so I don't have to worry about the kinds of problems other group members struggle with because I am in His hands." The patient might use age, if that is the distinguishing characteristic, to decide that the kinds of problems she has are so vastly different from those of the rest of the group, they could not possibly understand. Or, as in the case just described, the patient might decide that the group is not knowledgeable or sophisticated enough to help her.

The therapist must bear in mind that the ways in which the patient sees herself as a special case are motivated by anxiety. By agreeing to join the group in the first place, she has made it clear that there are issues in common. However, once in the group, anxiety mounts, overriding the gut sense that she needs help and support in coping with the disease, thereby causing her to establish distance from the group. Because anxiety is at the root of attempts to distance oneself, the first goal is to support the patient in an effort to quell the anxiety. By listening carefully to this member, the therapist can reinforce the similarities between herself and other members. The main strategy is to help the patient tolerate the anxiety and to connect with the rest of the group. By joining the group in this shared journey of self-exploration and mutual support, the patient will feel less isolated and able to face her particular fears and concerns in the context of a supportive and caring environment.

THE HELP REJECTOR

The help rejector is someone who insists that she is looking for help, if only she could find someone competent enough to give it to her. No one in the group, neither the members nor the leaders, can ever provide her with quite what she needs. Embedded in every reply she gives to others' responses to her appeals for help is a "Yes, but."

This member may believe her problems are so complicated and difficult that there is really nothing that can be done for her. Underlying this belief that her problems are too complex is often some reason for why she really does not want things to change in her life. One possibility is that she receives gratification from being someone perpetually in need of help. After all, if she took the advice given to her, perhaps her problems would be solved and there would be no one left to give her the sympathy and support she craves. Alternatively, the intricacy of her problems may be her way of establishing a sense of superiority. Underlying this need to feel better than the rest of the group are feelings of inadequacy and inferiority. By rejecting the help of others, she can keep people mystified and stymied about how to help her. The inscrutability of her needs is a way of keeping people from getting close enough to know her and, as she fears, see her inadequacies.

Rejecting help can also be a way of expressing anger. She may be feeling enraged at the unwarranted blow that life has dealt her. Her anger is preventing her from seeing any way to improve her life now or in the future. What may really be fueling the anger, however, is her fear that all is hopeless for her. What is the point in thinking anything can help her when she knows/fears that all is lost?

The task for the therapist is to bypass her rejection of help in order to access the underlying feeling. Such a patient is working hard to maintain her distance from others and her own feelings. It takes a sensitive and empathic orientation to help her soften so that she can attend to what is really going on inside of her. For example, following one of her rejections, the therapist might say, "While you were saying that, I was struck with how sad you looked. Is that how it feels to you?" The therapist must strive to "hear" what the patient is really asking, and to support her. Ignoring *what* she says and responding to *how* she says it may enable her to speak from a more authentic place.

Another approach is to remark on the fact that the group does not seem to be giving her what she needs or wants. "It seems that we are not able to give you the feedback you are seeking. What would you like from the group right now?" While she might not be able to say immediately or directly what it is that she needs, it can begin the process of enlisting her in the process of determining how the group can be most helpful.

Paradoxically, the help rejector is someone in need of a lot of help. Not only does she need help in coping with her cancer but she also needs help in maintaining relationships with others. She is trying to push people away and is often quite successful at it. The leader must be careful that she not become alienated from the group. When the help rejector rebuffs another member's suggestion, it is often useful to ask the member how it feels to have her advice rejected. Initially this can be threatening to both members, but it will enable the help rejector to respond to the other member as a person rather than another piece of advice she must fend off. When we help this woman "join" the group, she will benefit from the support she receives and the group will benefit from having supported her.

THE PSYCHIATRICALLY DISTRESSED

Cancer has no respect for age, race, socioeconomic status, education level, geography, or gender. Thus, there is no reason to think it would not cut across personalities. Although you can expect your cancer groups to be composed of well-functioning men and women, there is always the possibility of having in your group someone who has a history of psychiatric problems. These problems can include depression, anxiety disorders, mood disorders, personality disorders, drug abuse and psychosis.

Ideally, the group leaders will have assessed each potential member for psychiatric problems during the initial interview, and those who were clearly inappropriate for a supportive-expressive group would be referred elsewhere. But even with the initial screening, occasionally there will be someone with special needs who has joined the group. The leaders should try to attend to these needs as much as possible without disrupting the group. The task of the therapist is twofold: to be responsive to the special needs of each patient while keeping in mind the overall needs of the rest of the group.

It is important to create as supportive an environment as possible, partly by helping other members provide support for the patient. The therapist should remember, however, that for some disorders there exists a bottomless pit that no amount of group support could ever fill. The leaders should be alert to this possibility and not allow the group to become depleted by or resentful of the person's neediness.

If attempts to support the patient do not help the situation, it may be appropriate to recommend that the patient receive individual assessment and treatment in addition to the group. If it becomes clear that the special difficulties of this patient cannot be managed in the group and are disruptive, she may need to be removed from the group and referred for individual therapy.

When this type of situation arises, it is important to speak privately with the distressed patient and to be both empathic and honest. Discuss your observations about the patient's struggles and concerns. This might involve stating that you recognize a strong need for attention but that you are concerned that, because of the intensity with which this need is expressed, the patient will, in fact, get just the opposite. Elicit the patient's perspective on this issue. The aim of the discussion is to find a common understanding about what problems are beyond the scope of the group. Once this understanding is reached, you can begin talking about the additional resources the patient might have available to help her. By the end of the meeting, there should be a mutual agreement about appropriate expectations for what the group can offer, what issues are beyond the scope of the group, and where the patient might go to meet those needs. Be prepared to offer appropriate referrals.

THE HOSTILE MEMBER

Carrie was attending her first meeting in one of our long-standing metastatic breast cancer groups and got off to a quick start discussing her treatment and complaining that her doctors had consistently misdiagnosed her. She expressed considerable anger and in a somewhat righteous and preachy manner she dismissed the value of a positive attitude and warned the women about how little doctors care. "Your doctor will not be at your funeral, so you'd better make the decisions yourself." She clearly was having a negative effect on many of the members. She opined that men were different from women, because men were simply less empathic and more competitive. This appeared to be a clear dig at the male group leader and elicited much head shaking around the room. Carrie had made her grand entrance, which had everyone else looking for the exit door.

The therapist gently took up her challenge: "I hear that you don't like doctors in general and male doctors in particular. But are you here to fix me or get help for yourself?"

Surprisingly, Carrie's hostility, which she wore like a badge that first day, was the front behind which hid a frightened little girl. Difficult though she could be, Carrie was someone who could be reached, and her hostility could melt away. Because she had this potential to exude hostility, and even though several members grew to love her as one would a frightened and angry little girl, the relationship to Carrie was always ambivalent. In the end, she became very attached to the group and benefited enormously from their love and generosity. They were the family she never had and remained so until her death a year later.

The hostile member is perhaps the most dangerous member to have in a group. She has the potential to destroy feelings of safety and consequently can completely derail the group process.

It is important to distinguish between hostility and anger. Anger is both acceptable and expectable. People who have been diagnosed with cancer have reason to be angry. Anger is a healthy response, particularly when it is attached to the appropriate target. Certainly, problems can emerge if the anger is directed at the wrong target, especially if it is another group member. However, if it is purely misdirected anger and not hostility, then it is a matter of helping the patient identify what the anger is in response to and to help her direct the anger accordingly. This type of group work can be enormously helpful to everyone.

Hostility, on the other hand, is a destructive force. Hostile individuals seek to hurt others, often because they themselves have been seriously wounded. Isolated acts of hostility can be worked with, as long as the patient is able to recognize (with group help) the underlying need that is fueling the hostile behavior. However, it is the hostile individual who lacks insight about the hostility, who lacks remorse for the hostility, and who lacks the willingness to examine the hostility who is a real danger to the group and needs to be removed. Our recommendation is to not invite such individuals to participate in the group or to ask them to leave if the hostility becomes apparent after they have joined the group.

WHEN MEMBERS LEAVE

Occasionally a member will decide to leave the group. This can occur for any number of reasons. Two of the more common are that she is not getting her needs met, or that the group is too frightening. In any case, it is important that the reasons for leaving be determined and, if possible, addressed in the group before the person leaves. The decision to leave may reflect the patient's own issues; however, more often than not it is also a reflection of the group. This does not necessarily mean that there is something "wrong" with the group, but it may very well indicate that there is something in the group that needs to be addressed. Whatever the case, bringing the patient's reasons for leaving out into the open will provide the opportunity for all members to examine whether or not they are getting what they need from the group.

The decision to leave may be because there is someone else in the group who is demanding too much attention or derailing the focus of the group. This kind of situation can occur if it is a psychologically heterogeneous group—that is, where some members are psychologically healthier while others are more vulnerable and in need of more attention. If this is the situation, it is important that the problem be addressed because it is bound to be affecting other members as well.

Some individuals will leave because they find it too threatening to talk about cancer and how it has affected them. Before a member leaves for this reason, it is important to talk about how the discussions have affected her. Raising this issue with the group provides an occasion to address the fear and anxiety that is generated for all members when talking about various cancer-related topics. These fears and anxieties should be acknowledged as valid and real, but at the same time the leader can use this situation as an opportunity to reiterate the philosophy of these groups—that we believe the best way to cope with fear and anxiety about cancer is to talk about all the ways in which people are affected by it.

When a member tells you that she has decided to leave the group, your first response should be to inquire about the reasons. "Gwen, can you tell us what brought you to this decision?" Obviously, there can be a host of reasons that people can give for why they want to leave. Upon hearing the reason, inquire, or facilitate a discussion, about whether it is possible to address the reason for wanting to leave so that it is no longer a reason. The assumption is that there are obstacles—either psychological or practical—that are making it difficult for the person to continue. Your goal is to attempt to identify them and to remove them. This might involve reassuring the person that her feelings are both natural and to be expected or it might involve having the group discuss ways in which the group needs to change. However, if her reason for leaving is because her goals are incompatible with those of the group, then it is important to acknowledge that and accept it.

The main principle in dealing with a member's decision to leave is to face it head-on. If there are problems in the group, they ought to be addressed. If a member's leaving is not a reflection of the group, it still provides an opportunity to acknowledge the fear and anxiety with which each person struggles.

Finally, whenever anyone decides to leave, every effort should be made to have the member return for one last session so that the member and the other group members can say good-bye. This is important for all concerned as it is a message of caring. It is also a message that no one will slip away unnoticed.

CONCLUSION

In this chapter we have identified some challenging situations and individuals you might encounter when leading a supportive-expressive therapy group. Although problems that arise in groups are often difficult, they usually bring with them both danger and opportunity. The danger is that the problem will not be handled well and will in some way damage the group. The opportunity is that the problems bring with them the potential for growth, either in the individual with the problem, the group as a whole, or the group leaders. While it was not possible to discuss all types of problems that you might encounter, we hope that we have provided you with a way to conceptualize potential problems and with strategies that you can use and adapt to meet any challenge that arises.

CHAPTER 11

Methods of Pain Control

Pain is a common and annoying problem. It is the embodiment of both physical and mental discomfort, since it is not only unpleasant but is also an apparently inescapable reminder that something is wrong with your body.

Simple pain-control techniques using self-hypnosis can be quite effective in reducing or sometimes even eliminating pain (Hilgard and Hilgard, 1975; Spiegel and Bloom, 1983a; Patterson, Everett et al., 1992; Spiegel, 1991; Hilgard and LeBaron, 1982; Chaves, 1994; Holroyd, 1996). Cancer patients and others with pain are quickly able to learn, either individually or in groups, how to produce a combination of physical relaxation and control over attention that can help them to reduce substantially the amount of pain that they experience. As you sit reading this page, you are hopefully unaware of the sensations in your back, bottom, and legs touching the chair—at least until we remind you of them. Then, suddenly, they enter awareness, only to depart almost as quickly as you read the next sentence. We focus attention toward and away from sensations constantly, and patients can be taught to do the same—even with pain.

Most people with chronic pain come to realize that there are certain times when the pain seems to be worse—usually evenings and weekends, when there is less going on in the way of natural distractions from the pain sensations. Absorption in work or play is a natural analgesic. Diving into a project may seem such a welcome relief that we do it naturally and yet do not credit this redirection of our attention with its pain-relieving properties. In part this is because the minute we think about pain, we tend to feel it. Just being aware of pain tends to exacerbate it.

In pain-relief exercises, it is important that patients not misinterpret the discussion to imply that the pain is all in their heads. Pain is always a combination of physical and reactive distress. The fact that techniques such as hypnosis facilitate pain reduction does not imply that the pain is not real. Rather it underscores the patient's ability to enhance control over their own response to the pain. It is useful to take a rehabilitative approach to analgesia, encouraging patients to make the most of new opportunities to improve pain relief, rather than assuming that they are simply going to fix some emotional problem that causes pain.

REDUCING MUSCLE TENSION AND
DIVERTING ATTENTION FROM PAIN

Group members as well as patients in the individual setting can be taught some simple exercises to relieve tension, which will also help them to better understand and control pain:

Tension and Pain

1. Make a tight fist, tensing all the muscles in your forearm and upper arm. Now make it twice as tight—hard as you can. You should, by now, be feeling some discomfort in the normal muscles of your arm and hand. Now let go.

Lesson number 1: Muscle tension causes pain. You can produce painful sensations in a non-injured part of your body simply by tensing your muscles. And yet, what do most people with chronic pain do? They splint the part of the body that hurts, thereby producing tension in normal muscles and pulling on the part that hurts. This causes a natural but unwelcome increase in pain sensation.

Attention and Pain

2. Squeeze the webbing between the thumb and index finger of one hand with the thumb and index finger of the other hard enough that it hurts. See how much it does hurt. Now, think of the name of your second-grade schoolteacher. Now, let go.

You have just done a little experiment: You had the same physical discomfort in two conditions—first when you were paying full attention to it, and then while you were thinking about something else. If you are like most people, you had more pain in the first condition, when you were paying attention to it. Occasionally, someone feels more pain in the second condition, especially if they had a particularly bad second-grade schoolteacher.

Lesson number 2: You have to pay attention to pain for it to hurt. All pain is a product of the physical discomfort that triggers signals from the body, and the amount of conscious attention you pay to those signals is a major determinant of how much pain you feel. "The strain in pain lies mainly in the brain" (Spiegel and Spiegel, 1987, p. 262).

These exercises suggest that you can do several things to reduce pain simply by (1) reducing the amount of muscle tension that may increase the physical component of pain; and (2) increasing control over your attention so that you focus away from pain sensations.

The success of these techniques does not mean that the pain is not real. None would seriously claim that childbirth is not painful. Nonetheless, women have, for millennia, learned to produce children while modulating their physical discomfort. They experience real physical pain, but they can learn—by focusing on their breathing, looking at a spot, and staying in touch with their partner/coach—to reduce the discomfort caused by the stretching and contraction of their muscles in the birthing process. Using such techniques does not imply that the pain is not real. Rather, it indicates motivation to allow the pain to interfere minimally with your life.

REDUCING DEPRESSION AND
PAIN AND INTERPRETING PAIN

There are other factors besides muscle tension and attention that affect pain. It has been known for some time that depression and pain interact. People in pain seem more depressed, and depressed people complain more of pain (Hendler, 1984; Massie and Holland, 1990; Wells, Stewart et al., 1989; Spiegel, Sands et al., 1994; McDaniel and Nemeroff, 1993; Spiegel and Bloom, 1983b). Indeed, the original thinking was that people with various emotional disorders tended to complain more in general, and about pain in particular. The idea was that because they were anxious and depressed, these individuals made more of a fuss about pain, thereby amplifying it. More recently, an alternative point of view has emerged, suggesting that the experience of having chronic pain may make someone depressed (Hendler, 1984; Spiegel, Sands et al., 1994).

Depression is more than mere sadness or grief, loss or regret. It involves both mental and physical symptoms. Mentally depressed people tend to be excessively guilt-ridden and self-critical. They ruminate endlessly about past failures, blame themselves inappropriately for real or imagined short-comings, and ignore positive aspects of themselves. They feel hopeless, helpless, and worthless. They believe that there is little hope for improvement in the future, that there is little they can do to change their lot, and that they are worth very little. At times they contemplate or even attempt suicide. Physically depressed individuals have little energy, often sleep poorly, typically waking early in the morning unable to get back to sleep, and report little appetite or sexual energy. Such serious or major depression is not uncommon, affecting some 4 percent of the U.S. population at any one time (Myers, Weissman et al., 1984).

We became suspicious that the experience of chronic pain could indeed induce depression. We looked for factors that were associated with reports of pain among the breast cancer patients involved in our original support group study. We found three variables that were significantly associated with the intensity of their pain (Spiegel and Bloom, 1983b).

1. *Use of pain medications.* This meant that these patients, like many cancer patients, were undermedicated for their pain. Were they receiving adequate analgesic medication, there would either be no relationship, or even an inverse relationship between medication use and pain (i.e., the more medication taken, the less the pain). What seems to happen instead is that doctors are afraid that their patients will abuse pain medication or develop tolerance to it. Tolerance means that the same amount of pain medication produces less of an analgesic effect, leading to increasing doses and possible habituation or addiction. Alternatively, many patients are wary of taking such medications, being fearful of addiction, or more common side effects of sedation, loss of energy, or constipation. "I prefer to think in torment than not to be able to think at all," wrote Freud, who suffered during the last years of his life with cancer of the mouth, and who disliked pain medications.

Yet, as a group, cancer patients do not become drug abusers, and concerns about this are seriously exaggerated. The main problem is that, effective as modern analgesic medications are, they are on the one hand not a panacea and on the other are not widely or well enough utilized. They do not always work (especially if underprescribed), and they do have significant side effects. However, analgesic medication complements but does not replace the importance of psychological pain control techniques.

2. *Mood disturbance.* We found that those breast cancer patients who rated themselves as being more anxious and depressed on a formal rating scale called the Profile of Mood States, or POMS (McNair, Lorr et al., 1992), turned out to have more pain. As in previous studies, there was an apparent reinforcing effect of anxiety and depression with pain. We are finding a similar relationship between mood disturbance and pain in our current studies with metastatic breast cancer patients. In a recent study (Spiegel, Sands et al., 1994) we sought to better understand this relationship between depression and cancer. We recruited two samples of cancer patients, one with substantial pain, and one with very little pain, and intensively assessed them. We found, as you might expect, substantial differences in depression in the two samples. Indeed, 28 percent of those with substantial pain met criteria for major depression, the most serious kind, versus only 6 percent of the low-pain patient group. But, of even more interest is the fact that a previous history of major depression was far more common in the low-pain group. Thus, by history alone, they were the ones who should have been more vulnerable to depression. Yet, it was the high-pain patients who had it, leading us to the conclusion that pain produces depression. Rather than indicating that depressed people exaggerate pain, we conclude that pain makes people depressed, and this, in turn, makes it harder for them to tolerate the pain they have. Thus, a downhill cycle is produced, in which, as pain makes people more depressed, they tolerate the pain more poorly, become even more depressed, and so on.

There are good treatments available for depression, both antidepressant medications, and psychotherapies aimed at correcting depressive thoughts, and managing the emotional and interpersonal problems associated with depression (Elkin, Shea et al., 1989; Public Health Service, 1993; McDaniel, Musselman et al., 1995; Beck, Rush et al., 1979; Beck, 1995). These treatments can, in turn, reduce pain.

If a patient in a group shows signs that her depressive symptoms are increasing, particularly seeming to feel more helpless, overwhelmed, or worthless, the therapist should recommend an individual psychiatric evaluation. Sadness is not uncommon in such groups; it is when the depressed mood is pervasive and the patient feels undeserving of help and unable to respond to offers of assistance that further help may be needed. As mentioned earlier, depressed patients often make others angry because of their refusal to take others up on offers of help, as well as their tendency to see any situation as worse than it is. Also, suicidal ideation is a clear indication of the need for referral, evaluation, and treatment. The rates of major depression increase from 3 to 4 percent in the general population (Myers, Weissman et al., 1984) to 6 percent among the medically ill (Katon and Sullivan, 1990), 20 percent among those with terminal illness, and 60 percent among those who request assisted suicide (Chochinov, Wilson et al., 1995). Thus as the severity of medical illness increases, the likelihood of depression does as well. Group support is effective in reducing some but not all depressive symptoms (Spiegel, Bloom et al., 1981), so therapists must be alert to patients who are not responding and who may need more intensive and multimodal assistance.

3. *The meaning of pain.* To the extent that our breast cancer patients thought that pain signaled a worsening of the disease, they were more likely to report greater pain intensity.

Anesthesiologist Henry Beecher returned from his World War II combat experience on the Anzio beachhead in North Africa puzzled by his experiences there (Beecher, 1956). His main job in combat had been stopping bleeding and administering morphine for pain to wounded soldiers. He stopped a lot of bleeding, but noted that he had very few requests for morphine, even from very seriously injured soldiers. After the war he tried an experiment. We went to a group of civilian surgical patients at the Massachusetts General Hospital who were equally or less seriously injured than his soldiers, and asked if they wanted morphine for their pain. They insisted on medication. Thus, despite less serious injuries, they reported substantially more pain. Beecher concluded, correctly, that the meaning of pain influences its intensity. To a combat soldier, being alert with a wound meant you were likely to get out of the war alive, and you wanted to remain alert to make sure you got off the battlefield in one piece. To a civilian, the surgery and associated pain was just a threat to life, and therefore less tolerable and more painful.

Indeed, in our study (Spiegel and Bloom, 1983b) the site of metastasis did not significantly predict the amount of pain. It is reported that cancer which has spread to bones or organs produces more pain than that in soft tissue (Watson and Evans, 1982). Yet this was not the case in our study, and others have shown that the majority of identifiable metastatic lesions do not pro-duce pain (Front, Schneck et al., 1979). Indeed, contrary to popular belief, cancer is not uniformly associated with pain. Only about one-third of pa-tients with primary cancer report pain, and even among those with ad-vanced cancer that has spread to other parts of the body, only two out of three report significant pain (Bonica, 1979, 1990).

One means by which group therapy can help with pain is discussion of anxieties related to disease progression. Patients who are given the opportu-nity to express and explore their fears about disease progression are less likely to remind themselves of their anxiety by focusing on pain progression (Weisenberg, Aviram et al., 1984). Thus group discussions regarding fears of disease progression and death should help to relieve the signal function of pain and prevent it from triggering an escalating spiral of pain and anxiety.

Also, some individuals are more sensitive to pain than others, or are more likely to find it distressing—those with what is often referred to as a lower pain threshold. Again this does not mean they manufacture pain, but rather that they are more disturbed by it. However, this sensitivity is a double-edged sword—studies have shown that the people who complain more about headache pain, for example, are more likely to benefit from techniques such as hypnosis and biofeedback (Andreychuk and Skriver, 1975). Thus whatever cognitive and emotional factors may amplify pain due to anxiety and depression may also be utilized to diminish it.

There are numerous other techniques that can be helpful in controlling pain, ranging from yoga (Garfinkel, Singhal et al., 1998) to meditation train-ing (Kabat-Zinn, 1994) to guided imagery (Lyles, Burish et al., 1982; Lam-bert, 1996). They combine principles similar to those employed in teaching self-hypnosis, but in varying formats. They include methods designed to produce physical relaxation and control over the deployment of attention. They are often taught as courses. The advantage of self-hypnosis is that it is brief and can be introduced as just one portion of an overall group therapy program. In our protocol each group session ends with approximately five minutes of self-hypnosis. There is evidence that a given individual's capac-ity to experience hypnosis, or hypnotizability, which is a very stable trait (Hilgard, 1965; Spiegel and Spiegel, 1987), is correlated with the person's re-sponse to a variety of pain treatments, those explicitly employing hypnosis (Hilgard and Hilgard, 1975) and even those utilizing acupuncture (Katz, Kao et al., 1974; Moore and Berk, 1976; Knox and Shum, 1977).

TEACHING HYPNOSIS IN
THE GROUP SETTING

Hypnosis is a simple and natural form of focused attention that most people can use to filter out awareness of many kinds of pain and other discomforts. Hypnosis has three main components: absorption, dissociation, and suggestibility (Spiegel and Spiegel, 1987; Maldonado and Spiegel, 1996; Spiegel and Maldonado, 1999).

1. *Absorption* is a state of completely involved and self-altering attention, such as being so caught up in a good movie, novel, or play that you lose awareness of your surroundings and focus entirely on the imagined activity. Many individuals have had the experience of needing to reorient themselves after watching a good movie, or they may become so absorbed in a sunset or an idea that they ignore someone calling for them. This is a spontaneous hypnotic-like experience. Research shows that individuals who frequently have such absorbing experiences are more highly hypnotizable on formal testing (Tellegen and Atkinson, 1974).

2. *Dissociation* is an ability to separate or compartmentalize aspects of memory, identity, or consciousness that would ordinarily be processed together (APA, 1994; Spiegel and Cardeña, 1991; Spiegel, 1997; Maldonado and Spiegel, 1998). The example given at the beginning of the chapter of ignoring sensations in one's body until they are called to your attention is an example of everyday dissociation. Other examples include the experience of discovering an injury—finding a cut or a bruise—with no memory of how it happened.

Indeed, there is growing evidence that people frequently respond to trauma with dissociation (Marmar, Weiss et al., 1994; Bremner, Southwick et al., 1992; Cardeña and Spiegel, 1993; Spiegel, Hunt et al., 1988; Yehuda, Elkin et al., 1996; Koopman, Classen et al., 1994). They spontaneously use it as a way to distance themselves emotionally from physical discomfort and extreme anxiety.

A petite young woman who suffered from Hodgkin's disease, a cancer of the lymphatic system (white blood cells), proved to be very hypnotizable, and learned quickly to control her persistent nausea and vomiting from chemotherapy with self-hypnosis. She simply imagined that she was on vacation, enjoying the beach rather than being in the chemotherapy infusion room.

A psychiatrist was interviewing her about her successful use of this technique in front of some psychiatric residents, and, by way of taking a routine history, asked her if she had ever been hospitalized before.

"Yes," she replied. "I broke my pelvic bone when I fell off of a third-story balcony." My God, she was suicidal and must have jumped, and I missed it, he thought. "Did you jump?" he asked. "No," she answered, "I was pushed." By this point he had concluded that she was paranoid. "What do you mean?" he asked.

"I was standing on a balcony next to this huge, beefy guy with a beer in his hand. He turned around suddenly and just knocked me over the edge of the balcony. It was a stupid accident." Feeling upset at the thought of the sudden fall, the psychiatrist summoned his most empathic tone, and said, "That must have been terrifying." "No," she replied, "it was quite pleasant." By this time he knew she must be psychotic. But he was wrong. "Let me tell you how I experienced it. I felt as if I were standing on another balcony watching a pink cloud float down to the ground. I felt no pain at all, and even tried to walk back up-stairs." She had spontaneously used her remarkable dissociative ability to distance herself from the fear and pain that would normally be associated with such an injury.

Dissociation is a natural complement to the absorption that typifies the hypnotic state (Spiegel and Spiegel, 1987). The more engrossed you are in one central object of attention, the more likely you are to ignore others. Thus the price paid for intensity of focus is the displacement from conscious awareness of whole portions of consciousness, and the greater context surrounding perception.

3. *Suggestibility.* There is a common fear that, once hypnotized, a person is deprived of will and choice, and can be made to do anything. It is certainly not the case that a hypnotized person is unable to make choices or to refuse to do something. On the other hand, there is something to hypnotic suggestibility, in that in a hypnotic state people are less likely to break with a suggestion because they are less likely to think it over (Spiegel, 1974; Spiegel and Spiegel, 1987; Hilgard, 1991). When we are in a state of mind that emphasizes focusing on the content of an idea, we are less likely to evaluate it or the person who suggested it. We have all had the experience of wondering how on earth we went along with someone and did something that in retrospect seemed unwise. "It seemed like a good idea at the time" is what we usually tell ourselves. Another price of hypnotic absorption is of a suspension of critical judgment, a willingness to immerse oneself in the *what* rather than the *why* of a situation. This allows you to do more but to reflect on it less.

HYPNOSIS AND MIND/BODY CONTROL

There are at least three ways in which entering such an altered mental state as hypnosis may be helpful in controlling mind/body interactions:

1. *The state itself.* It may be that there is something inherently useful about being in a trancelike state from time to time. It seems to be a kind of relaxed attention, allowing for a comfortable state of alertness. Such a state may help you examine problems without the associated physical tension, making it possible to deal with problems without their seeming so overwhelming.

Betty, whom we discussed earlier, came for a consultation not primarily because of her breast cancer, but rather because her husband had just been diagnosed with Alzheimer's disease, a relentlessly progressive dementia that leads to loss of memory, of other cognitive abilities, and of physical control, and eventually to death. She was overwhelmed with misery. She had just come to terms with her own cancer, which was a worry but had not spread, and had been planning a happy period of retirement and freedom to pursue creative activities. Now she felt imprisoned by her life, unable to escape the endless worries that beset her.

Her concerns were real and understandable, but the therapist tried to help her see them from a different point of view. In hypnosis, she pictured one of her concerns on an imaginary screen, as though she were watching a home video, with the rule that no matter what she saw on the screen, she would maintain a physical sense of floating relaxation in her body. She cried as she saw an image of her beloved husband deteriorating. She was then asked to divide the screen in half, and picture something she might do about the problem on the other side. She had been quite resentful of her sister's unwillingness to help her deal with previous common family problems. She began to formulate a plan for eliciting more help from her sister and other members of the family.

Another technique was also tried. She was told to use the hypnosis as though she were looking through a camera with a telephoto and a wide-angle lens. She could thus make what she was looking at bigger or smaller, either focusing on it intensely or placing it in a broader context. She was intrigued by this, finding a sense of emotional relief in being able to play with the size of the problem. She emerged from the hypnosis with a tear-stained face, but noticed that she did not feel quite as overwhelmed by her problems: "I realize that there is more to me than my problems, bad as they are."

2. *Shifting between states.* There may be something healthful about the alternation among mental states. We know, for example that it is not only refreshing but necessary to alternate between sleep and wakefulness each day.

Restorative processes occur in sleep that help the brain function better during wakefulness. Sleep researcher Alan Hobson (Hobson and Stickgold, 1995) has shown that there is a shift in the dominance of neurotransmitter activity in sleep toward the neurons that secrete acetylcholine, with a relative shutdown of the nerves that produce the alerting neurotransmitters epinephrine and norepinephrine, which are secreted in large amounts during "fight or flight" reactions. Thus sleep provides for restoration of depleted arousal neurotransmitters, as others take over.

It may well be that the cyclic alternation between normal and trancelike states in consciousness serves a similar restorative function, allowing not only for a change in cognitive or emotional appraisal of a difficult situation, but for restoration of mental energy.

3. *Special advantages of the hypnotic state.* There is evidence that people in hypnotic states have unusually good control over physical processes (Spiegel and Vermetten, 1993). It has been clearly demonstrated, for example, that hypnosis can be used as part of an effective treatment for warts (Ewin, 1992; Spanos, Stenstrom et al., 1988; Spanos, Williams et al., 1990; Surman, Gottlieb et al., 1973; Sinclair-Gieben and Chalmers, 1959). Patients given a hypnotic suggestion that their warts will go away will lose them at a much faster rate than control subjects who have not been given such hypnotic suggestions. Similarly, hypnosis has been used effectively to induce or eliminate allergic skin reactions, treat other skin conditions such as psoriasis (Frankel, 1987), and control skin blood flow and temperature (Maslach, Marshall et al., 1972). Highly hypnotizable individuals can produce a difference in the temperature of their hands of as much as 4 degrees centigrade in just a few minutes, simply by imagining in hypnosis that one is warm (in the sun or in a warm bath) and the other is cold (in snow or ice).

Hypnosis has also been used to facilitate treatment of disorders of the digestive system, such as irritable bowel syndrome, in which people suffer chronic abdominal distention, discomfort, and diarrhea (Whorwell, Prior et al., 1984, 1987). It has also been effectively used to help people with asthma, those subject to sudden attacks of wheezing because of constriction of the bronchioles (Ewer and Stewart, 1986; Kohen, Olness et al., 1984; Morrison, 1988; Covino and Frankel, 1993). Asthmatics can learn to shift quickly into a simple state of self-hypnosis and reduce the anxiety-related physical tension that increases rather than decreases constriction in the lungs. There is evidence that those who are more highly hypnotizable are more likely to respond well to such treatments (Collison, 1975).

Given this evidence that hypnosis provides an opportunity for enhanced control over physical processes, the reader may well be wondering why we don't simply suggest that the cancer will recede, or be consumed by eager white blood cells acting like sharks and devouring them, as some have advised. The reason is that there is simply no evidence that this happens. Just because your ability to control physical processes may be increased in hypnosis does not mean that you have infinite power to fix things in the body just because you "fixed" them in the mind. While some may find that imagining that their body is fighting off the cancer effectively is emotionally reassuring in some way, it can and does lead some to blame themselves if the cancer progresses, feeling that they have not done a good enough job of visualizing.

> *A brilliant woman in our study who wrote books on computer programming decided to travel for a special program to learn a cancer visualization technique. When she returned, she was told by her oncologist that she had suffered a substantial spread of her disease in the interim. When she called her counselor from the visualization program back, the counselor asked her: "Why did you want your cancer to spread?"*

There is, in fact, evidence that such take-charge approaches do not have any effect on the course of disease progression (Morgenstern, Gellert et al., 1984; Gellert, Maxwell et al., 1993). Thus it is unfair to burden cancer patients with the expectation that they should be able to control the development of their illness through direct mental effort. This can make them feel unduly guilty, or saddle them with an inappropriate optimism that undermines the necessary process of anticipatory grief and goal reappraisal described earlier in this book.

Similarly, loved ones should also not be made to feel responsible for a patient developing cancer. A businesswoman from New York called to inquire about supportive resources for families of cancer patients. She had a seven-year-old son with leukemia, and had called a program for help. She was told: "Any child with cancer is an unwanted child." She then called us to ask for and receive reassurance that she had done nothing to cause her child's cancer.

At the same time, there is every reason to use whatever techniques we have at hand to help cancer patients control symptoms such as pain, anxiety, nausea, and vomiting. In our support groups, these techniques are carried out after hypnosis is formally induced.

Some find it helpful to establish a baseline for evaluating their pain, so that they can assess how effective these exercises are in reducing pain. Most people can rate their current pain on a scale from zero to ten, with ten being unbearable pain, the worst ever, and zero being none at all. You can ask patients to take a moment to rate their pain on a zero-to-ten scale.

HYPNOTIC ANALGESIA EXERCISE

A self-hypnosis exercise is a comforting and effective way to conclude group sessions. With about five minutes to go, the group is asked to prepare for this exercise. The principles of the hypnotic intervention are the following:

Hypnotic Induction

The hypnotic induction utilized is just a quick shift in attention. Patients are asked to look up, close their eyes, and turn inward. Since hypnosis is just a shift in attention, effective induction to the state can be made in a matter of seconds rather than minutes.

(a) Float

The next step is to induce a sense of physical relaxation by teaching patients to imagine and affiliate with a physical image that conveys (but does not directly suggest) relaxation, such as floating or buoyancy.

(b) Filter

Patients are taught to establish a psychological filter between themselves and the pain signals, to filter the hurt out of the pain. This approach does not rely on insisting that the pain (or the cancer) will go away, but rather by focusing on altering the sensation of the pain, and learning to separate that sensation from the suffering, or amount of discomfort it causes.

It helps to ask patients to remember what physical remedies give them relief from the pain. Some get real relief by taking a warm bath; others by putting ice or cold water on the part of their body that hurts. This can form the basis of an effective self-hypnotic image of taking a luxurious warm bath or, alternatively, surrounding the part of your body that hurts with ice or snow. Then patients are instructed to feel a sense of warm or cool tingling numbness penetrating deeper and deeper into the part of their body that hurts. This becomes a filter that can filter the hurt out of the pain. They thus learn to substitute the temperature change for the discomfort.

(c) Focus

For some people, sensations other than temperature work better. It may help them to imagine lightness, heaviness, tingling, or numbness. Others find that they are capable of more dramatic leaps of the imagination, and can picture themselves simply going somewhere else, taking an imaginary vacation to a place they enjoy or have always wanted to visit.

Marc is a world-class swimmer who collapsed in an alley one evening and was brought to the Emergency Room. It turned out that he had a lymphoma (a cancer of the white blood cells) the size of a grapefruit in his abdomen, and it had begun to bleed. He very nearly died that first evening, but was stabilized and admitted to the hospital, where he was begun on chemotherapy.

He was suffering considerable pain, to the point that he would literally bang on the walls, and the nurses found it too emotionally stressful to care for him. His parents were afraid that he was becoming a drug addict. At that point, a psychiatrist was summoned to see him.

First, the psychiatrist reassured his parents that drug addiction was the least of his problems. When he saw Marc, he was lying in bed, groaning. "I bet you don't want to be here," he commented. "You spent years in medical school to figure that out?" Marc replied. The psychiatrist assessed his hypnotizability and, finding him hypnotizable, taught him to enter a state of self-hypnosis. He then asked him, as he continued to groan and writhe, where he would rather be. "I'm a great swimmer, but I've never surfed," he replied. "Good," the psychiatrist said, "we're going to Hawaii." Marc continued groaning, but soon there was a slightly different tone to his groans. "What happened?" the psychiatrist asked. "I fell off the surfboard," he replied. "Good. This time, get on it and do it right," insisted the psychiatrist. He had him practice this self-hypnosis "surfing" exercise every one to two hours, and any time the pain got bad.

Within forty-eight hours, Marc was off of all his pain medications, and was joking with the nurses, chasing them up and down the halls in his bear-claw slippers. The attending physician's note in the chart read: "Patient off of pain meds. Tumor must be regressing."

(d) Forget

For others, distraction works better. They can learn to simply concentrate on sensations in other, nonpainful parts of their body. They can be instructed to attend to, for example, the delicate sensations in their fingertips as they rub them together. They learn to notice how pleasant and interesting those sensations can feel, and concentrate on them when they are tempted to focus on the pain.

Getting to the pain early is an important principle in pain management. It is far easier to interrupt an attack of pain before it gets established than to reduce severe pain that has been causing discomfort for some time. This is true of pharmacologic and well as psychological interventions. It seems that a feedback pathway gets set up once pain begins that makes it more difficult, though not impossible, to interrupt. It is thus wise to advise patients to practice their self-hypnosis regularly, and to use it at the first indication of any increase in their pain.

Induction into Self-Hypnosis

The first step is to help the members enter a safe and comfortable state in which they are floating comfortably, and have focused their attention inward.

"Get as comfortable as you can. First, look straight ahead. Then look up to the top of your head. While looking up, close your eyes slowly. Take a deep breath, let your eyes relax but keep them closed, and let your body float.

Imagine your body floating somewhere safe and comfortable, just floating right down through the chair. You might imagine yourself floating in a bath, a lake, in the ocean, in a hot tub, or just floating in space. Feel that pleasant sense of your body floating, floating right down through the chair. Let each breath become deeper and easier, and let the tension flow out of your body with each breath out.

And if you are aware of any pain right now, imagine a sensation of warm or cold tingling numbness developing in that part of your body, and let it surround the pain. Feel the tingling numbness enveloping that part of your body. Feel the warmth or coolness as a protective filter, to filter the hurt out of the pain.

If you feel any discomfort now, imagine that this part of your body is becoming warmer or cooler, lighter or heavier, or is starting to tingle. Notice how you can place a protective filter of warm or cool tingling numbness between you and the pain. That's right, just filter the hurt out of the pain. Imagine rubbing snow on the part of your body that hurts, or taking a nice warm bath. Just filter the hurt out of the pain."

Situational Anxiety

Self-hypnosis can easily be adapted to many stressful situations that tend to provoke anxiety. One common example is modern diagnostic scanners, such as CAT (Computerized Axial Tomography) and MRI (Magnetic Resonance Imaging). These noninvasive techniques provide detailed images of the inside of the body, and are a remarkable advance over simple x-ray and invasive angiography (injecting radio-opaque dyes into blood vessels coupled with x-ray) used only a few years ago. Nonetheless, the techniques, although now physically quite safe, can be emotionally stressful. The patient is often required to lie in a tightly enclosed space for up to an hour or more.

MRI scanners are noisy, with a loud clanking sound. And, naturally, the patient is worried about what the scans will show: Has the disease progressed or not? Is the treatment working?

Just allow your body to float, and picture in your mind's eye an imaginary screen— a movie screen, a TV screen, or a piece of clear blue sky. As you let your body float here, just imagine that you are somewhere you enjoy being.

One woman was so afraid of her MRI scan that she kept refusing it. It was absolutely necessary, since she had a brain tumor that threatened to impinge on her spinal cord, and might at some time require surgery to prevent paralysis. With some assistance she made a creative use of the self-hypnosis exercise, imagining that the clanking of the MRI scanner was from a motorboat. She loved water skiing, and pictured herself being pulled along by a motorboat while the scan was being done. She found it surprisingly easy to undergo the test in this way.

There is now evidence that teaching patients self-hypnosis can reduce anxiety and pain, even when they are undergoing invasive procedures involving arterial access and injection of dyes, as well as intravascular procedures. In one randomized trial (Lang, Joyce et al., 1996), patients randomly assigned to this kind of support in addition to patient-controlled analgesia (analgesics administered through an in-dwelling intravenous line) used one-ninth the medication, had less than half the pain, and had fewer procedural interruptions. They even got out of the recovery room sooner.

CONTROLLING NAUSEA AND VOMITING

Unfortunately, modern chemotherapies have some uncomfortable side effects. Prominent among them are nausea and vomiting (Morrow and Morrell, 1982). A strange kind of association, known as classical conditioning, may be set up between the sights, smells, and sounds of the treatment environment and the feelings associated with treatment. If patients become nauseated after receiving chemotherapy, they learn to associate the place of treatment with the feelings of discomfort. Some patients find themselves feeling ill before receiving chemotherapy rather than after. At times just the sight, or smell, or even the thought of the treatment room may be enough to provoke an attack of nausea. These side effects are bad enough without psychological amplification.

One approach that is often helpful is to try to distance the patient emotionally from the treatment environment:

You have to deliver your body for treatment, but you do not have to be there. Ask the nurse or tech to let you rest quietly, lie down, close your eyes, and let your body float. After you have established that floating sensation, use your imaginary screen to picture yourself where you would rather be. It might a safe and comfortable room at home, a beautiful place in the mountains or by the sea, or some vacation spot you enjoy. Try picturing parts of the world you would like to see. You can play a little trick on the treatment team—leave your body here, while you go somewhere else.

In this way, many patients are able to disrupt the associations between the setting and the physical response to it, by imagining that they are somewhere else. One woman found that she tired of simply enjoying the view, and needed to involve herself in a productive task. She loved interior decorating, so she imagined that she had acquired an old castle on the Rhine, with some forty rooms. She spent her chemotherapy time decorating these imaginary rooms, one by one.

This exercise can be used in anticipation of the treatment sessions as well.

CONCLUSION

Simple changes in the way patients mentally approach some of the physical problems associated with cancer—pain, anxiety, and nausea and vomiting—can make a big difference. Pain tends to make patients feel helpless. Techniques like hypnosis, which supposedly reduce control, are actually effective mechanisms for teaching patients how to enhance their control over their bodies. Even a relatively minor modulation of pain can have a very positive effect on a patient's sense of efficacy in controlling it, and some can substantially reduce or eliminate it. Like rocks in a fast-moving river, the pain is there, but the comfort and enjoyment with which the patients may make their trip—equipped with tools to control emotional and physical pain—can powerfully influence the quality and course of their lives.

Afterword

We have reviewed the research literature and described the methods involved in providing supportive-expressive group therapy designed to help people facing life-threatening illness. Our experience over more than two decades convinces us that these techniques are reassuring and helpful to those who suffer the anxiety, sadness, physical discomfort, and social dislocation that come with cancer, HIV-infection, and other life-threatening illnesses. There is now a growing body of data that indicates that providing such support is helpful.

PSYCHOLOGICAL OUTCOME OF
SUPPORTIVE-EXPRESSIVE GROUP THERAPY

Our own randomized studies indicate that breast cancer patients offered this treatment become less distressed, while control patients do not. In our original intervention trial for metastatic breast cancer patients, scores on the Profile of Mood States (POMS) declined over the initial year of treatment for patients who received it, while mood disturbance increased among those who received only routine care (Spiegel, Bloom et al. 1981). In addition, treatment patients were coping better, using less denial and avoidance. This occurred despite the fact that one-third of the treatment sample died during the initial year, meaning that the overall improvement occurred during a period when group members were exposed to the dying and death of others in their groups. We also found that these women experienced only half as much pain by the end of the year as did control patients, indicating that the self-hypnosis they had been taught was quite helpful (Spiegel and Bloom, 1983a). In our current intervention trial with metastatic breast cancer patients, we have found again that participating in support groups reduces symptoms of distress, such as mood disturbance and posttraumatic stress symptoms (Classen, Butler et al., in submission).

Our recent work with women who have primary breast cancer is consistent with the metastatic breast cancer findings. In a multicenter trial involving eleven oncology practices in the Community Clinical Oncology Program of the National Cancer Institute, we found that initial mood disturbance in the POMS was reduced over the initial six months (Spiegel, Morrow et al., 1996). Results of a subsequent randomized trial indicated a significant reduction in mood disturbance for those patients who started out with high mood disturbance (Classen, Koopman et al., in submission). We have similar findings in our studies of HIV-infected individuals, with preliminary data showing significant reductions in POMS scores among men randomized to supportive-expressive group therapy. This finding is consistent with the work of Kelly and colleagues (Kelly, Murphy et al., 1993), who found that supportive-expressive group therapy for those with HIV led to symptom reduction.

These findings from our laboratory are consistent with the observations of other research groups on the effects of group support of various types for cancer patients. Lipsey and Wilson (1993) reported a meta-analysis of the efficacy of psychological, educational, and behavioral treatments for health-related problems and found effect sizes that ranged from 0.21 to 1.30, almost without exception. To illustrate the consistency and magnitude of these positive outcomes, they compared the effect sizes of these psychosocial interventions (grand mean of 0.47) with those of standard medical interventions for cancer, heart disease, and HIV infection. The biomedical effect sizes ranged from 0.08 to 0.47. The authors note limitations in such a comparison, given that there are major differences in population and outcome criteria and that even a small increment in survival is significant. Nonetheless, their analysis shows that even relatively modest effects of medical interventions are often given more weight than consistently positive effects of psychotherapeutic interventions on emotional outcome. Furthermore, even less attention has been paid to the combined efficacy of psychosocial and medical intervention, which is the way it should be done. The authors conclude: "On balance, therefore, the magnitude of effect size estimates that meta-analysis reveals for psychological treatment seems sufficiently large to support the claim that such treatment is generally efficacious in practical as well as statistical terms" (p. 1199).

Other authors have reached similar conclusions regarding the efficacy of group interventions for cancer patients (Fawzy, Fawzy et al., 1995). Despite variations in populations studied and methods employed, group psychotherapy seems to work. There are, however, contrary reports. Helgeson and colleagues (1999) recently reported that an educational program was superior to a supportive group intervention for primary breast cancer patients. Indeed, the combination of the two actually seemed to detract from the benefits of the educational program. It may be that in this trial, the brief supportive intervention was enough to stir up but not resolve emotional issues, therefore accounting for the poor outcome. More typical of the outcome literature are reports that group therapy reduces a variety of symptoms, including anxiety and depression (Ferlic, Goldman et al., 1979; Gustafson and Whitman, 1978; Wood, Milligan et al., 1978; Spiegel, Bloom et al., 1981), improves coping skills (Turns, 1988; Fawzy, Cousins et al., 1990), and reduces symptoms such as pain, nausea, and vomiting (Forester, Kornfeld et al., 1985; Cain, Kohorn et al., 1986; Morrow and Morrell, 1982; Spiegel and Bloom, 1983a).

Various types of psychosocial interventions have been studied. Some lasted only six weeks and have been shown to improve coping skills and mood among malignant melanoma patients (Fawzy, Cousins et al., 1990). Others have helped reduce pain, nausea, and vomiting (Forester, Kornfeld et al., 1985; Cain, Kohorn et al., 1986; Morrow and Morrell, 1982). In some studies, improvement in psychosocial functioning is observed at the end of the intervention (Telch and Telch, 1986), while in others more obvious effects of the intervention appear six months later (Fawzy, Kemeny et al., 1990; Fawzy, Cousins et al., 1990).

PREDICTORS OF RESPONSE TO TREATMENT

Those most in need of help are most likely to benefit from it when it is provided, and tend to persist in doing poorly without it. Initial levels of mood disturbance are strong predictors of subsequent distress (Ell et al., 1989). Predictors of good response to treatment are a history of depression (Maunsell, Brisson et al., 1992), low self-esteem (Felton, Revenson et al., 1984; Timko and Janoff-Bulman, 1985), external locus of control (Northouse and Swain, 1987), and neuroticism (Morris, Greer et al., 1977), as reviewed in Irvine, Brown et al. (1991). Those whose initial distress is greatest are likely to benefit most from psychotherapeutic intervention. This is our experience as well, especially among women with recently diagnosed breast cancer. However, as the severity of illness increases and the prognosis becomes poorer, the percentage of patients likely to benefit from group therapy gets larger.

The absence of social support should also predict greater need for intervention, since social support for women with breast cancer is associated with improved adjustment, emotional well-being, and reduced fear of recurrence (Irvine, Brown et al., 1991; Woods and Earp, 1978; Jamison, Wellisch et al., 1978; Northouse, 1981; Reynolds and Kaplan, 1990). Bloom (1982) demonstrated that social contact and perceived family cohesiveness directly improve coping and indirectly affect patient adjustment. Warmth, support, and reciprocity within families are associated with decreased depression, as well as better family functioning (Primomo, Yates et al., 1990). Thus groups may both directly provide additional emotional and social support, and indirectly encourage interaction, which will improve patients' use of their social resources. One unresolved problem for future research is the relative benefit of group support for those who have and those who lack good family and other social resources. While it may be that groups most help those who have little support elsewhere, it may also be that those who have assembled the best social support in their family and personal lives will also make the best use of group therapy—"Those who have, get." It could also be that each type of person will benefit, but in different ways, receiving quantity versus quality of support, for example.

MEDICAL TREATMENT ADHERENCE

Some have been concerned that joining support groups may somehow undermine medical treatment by causing patients to rely more on their support groups and therapists and less on their physicians. Our experience is to the contrary. Patients in our groups seem to work out better relationships with their doctors, and this spirit of collaboration improves rather than diminishes adherence to treatment. Others have observed the same thing (Hoagland, Morrow et al., 1983; Steckel, 1982; Richardson, Shelton et al., 1990). Educating patients about the efficacy of treatments produces better adherence with medication regimens (Ferguson and Bole, 1979).

Variables that are known to affect adherence include demographics; patient perceptions of their illness and their role in its treatment; social support; the costs and benefits of adherence from the patient's perspective; and an intention to comply (Given and Given, 1989). All of these psychosocial factors except demographics can be influenced by participating in a support group. Such group experience can increase patient knowledge and change attitudes about treatment and may help patients overcome practical obstacles to adherence. To the extent that groups help patients take an active and collaborative role in their medical treatment, they will be more satisfied with their treatment and will more fully participate in it (Eisenthal, Emery et al., 1979; Wyszynski, 1990). Thus there is reason to believe that participation in therapy groups will improve adherence by helping patients to (1) better manage the anxiety that is intertwined with treatment, (2) better understand the reasoning behind treatment decisions, (3) feel more in control of the course of treatment through clearer communication with their physicians, and (4) more effectively mobilize support from friends and family for participating in treatment.

EFFECTS OF GROUP SUPPORT
ON HEALTH OUTCOMES

Providing social support interventions for isolated individuals under stress has been related to improved health outcomes (Fawzy, 1991; Raphael, 1977; Richardson, Shelton et al., 1990; Rodin, 1980; Spiegel, Bloom et al., 1989; Turner, 1981). Stress, both acute and chronic, has been associated with a variety of adverse health outcomes (McEwen, 1998). Even chronic mild stressors may produce a cumulative effect that is damaging to mood via depression, and to the body via effects on autonomic, endocrine, and immune function. Social support has been shown to be an important factor in mediating individuals' ability to cope with stress. Rodin (Rodin, 1980, 1986) observed decreases in urinary free cortisol levels in geriatric patients exposed to education about stress management. Moreover, she found that subjects who received this experimental coping intervention were not only rated as happier and more sociable, but also had longer survival times than groups that were not treated. Forester and colleagues (1985) found that both mood disturbance and physical symptoms of anorexia, fatigue, and nausea and vomiting were significantly improved compared to those of a matched control group in a sample of forty-eight cancer patients.

Recent research has provided surprising evidence that group psychotherapy may affect health status and the quantity as well as the quality of life. Providing social support interventions particularly for isolated individuals under stress has been related to improved health outcome (Fawzy, Fawzy et al., 1993; Raphael, 1977; Richardson, Shelton et al., 1990; Rodin, 1980, 1986; Spiegel, Bloom et al., 1989; Turner, 1981). Social support seems to serve as a stress buffer, and thus may be an important factor in mediating individuals' ability to cope with stress.

There is evidence that participation in psychosocial group treatment for metastatic cancer patients doubles from the point of randomization, an average of eighteen months (Spiegel, Bloom et al., 1989). Differences in disease course were independent of any differences in medical treatment received (Kogon et al., 1997). Thus the longer survival time was not due to some difference in medical treatment offered or received.

Two other randomized trials have demonstrated a psychosocial effect on survival among cancer patients. Richardson and colleagues (1990) utilized a four-cell design among patients with lymphomas and leukemias. Patients were assigned either to a routine care condition or to one of three educational and home-visiting supportive interventions. The control group had significantly shorter survival time than patients allocated to the intervention. There were also differences in patients' adherence with medical treatment as measured by allopurinol intake. However, the survival differences held even when differences in medication adherence were controlled.

Fawzy and colleagues published psychosocial, immunological, recurrence, and survival results of a randomized trial involving eighty patients with malignant melanoma. Half were assigned to routine care and the other half to a structured series of twelve support groups. These weekly meetings were designed to help patients better cope with the illness and its effects on their families. Initially, Fawzy and colleagues (Fawzy, Cousins et al., 1990) found significant reductions in mood disturbance on the POMS and the use of more active coping strategies in the intervention sample. In a companion report (Fawzy, Kemeny et al., 1990), they observed significant differences in immune function at six-month follow-up but not earlier. They found a predicted increase in natural killer cytotoxicity and an increase in LEU56 cells in the intervention sample. A recent six-year follow-up (Fawzy, Fawzy et al., 1993) demonstrated significantly lower rates of melanoma recurrence and mortality among intervention patients, consistent with the findings among breast cancer patients in our laboratory.

Some studies show no effect of psychosocial treatment on medical outcome. The apparent beneficial effect of psychosocial support on survival time of thirty-four breast cancer patients in another study (Morgenstern et al., 1984) disappeared when time from cancer diagnosis to program entry was controlled. This lack of difference has recently been confirmed in a long-term follow-up of the same sample (Gellert, Maxwell et al., 1993). Three randomized trials also found no survival benefit to psychotherapy for cancer patients. Linn and colleagues (1982) offered individual psychotherapy to a group of patients with a variety of cancers, including those of the lung and pancreas. There was psychological benefit but no effect on survival time. It may be that since virtually all of the patients died during the follow-up year, their disease was too far advanced to be significantly influenced by the psychotherapeutic support. Similarly, Ilnyckyj and colleagues (1994) and Cunningham and colleagues (1998) found no survival advantage for breast cancer patients randomly assigned to one of several group psychotherapies, some peer-led. In neither study was there any demonstrable psychological benefit. Thus the relative inefficacy of the intervention may account for the lack of medical effect.

However, whether or not a supportive-expressive group intervention helps people live longer, the crucial issue is that it helps them live better. The treatment is not focused on conquering cancer or other medical illness, but rather on hoping for the best but preparing for the worst. One cannot honestly face existential issues while pretending to wish away cancer or being artificially certain of cheating death. The focus of this treatment is care rather than cure—living fully in the face of serious illness rather than avoiding or taming it. One patient joked with her group, "Am I living longer yet?" Whatever future data indicate about the effect of such group support on survival time, in any given group there will be no guarantee that the psychotherapy employed in that setting will extend patient survival time. The key focus of the group should be on how well rather than how long the patients live.

More research is clearly needed on such problems as what are the most crucial aspects of treatment, which patients are most likely to benefit, what training is most effective for therapists, and what are the benefits of supportive-expressive group therapy. At the same time, we have evidence of its efficacy, and of its effectiveness in a variety of settings. This treatment combines what we know about psychotherapy with the healing power of social support. We hope it illustrates how medical science can regain its balance of compassion and competence. There is power in numbers, both the kind that inform research, and in the convening of those with common problems to help one another.

References

American Psychiatric Association (APA) (1994). *American Psychiatric Association: Diagnostic and Statistical Manual of Mental Disorders*, 4th edition. Washington, DC: American Psychiatric Press.

Anderson, B. (1992). Psychological interventions for cancer patients to enhance the quality of life. *Journal of Consulting and Clinical Psychology* 60(4):552–568.

Andreychuk, T., and C. Skriver (1975). Hypnosis and biofeedback in the treatment of migraine headache. *International Journal of Clinical and Experimental Hypnosis* 23(3):172–183.

Baider, L., T. Peretz, and A. Kaplan De-Nour (1992). Effect of the Holocaust on coping with cancer. *Social Science and Medicine* 34(1):11–15.

Barraclough, J., C. Osmond, I. Taylor, M. Perry, and P. Collins (1993). Life events and breast cancer prognosis [letter; comment]. *British Medical Journal* 307(6899):325.

Barraclough, J., P. Pinder, M. Creddas, C. Osmond, I. Taylor, and M. Perry (1992). Life events and breast cancer prognosis [see comments]. *British Medical Journal* 304(6834):1078–1081.

Beck, A., A. Rush, B. Shaw, and G. Emery (1979). *Cognitive Therapy of Depression*. New York: Guilford Press.

Beck, J. S. (1995). Cognitive Therapy: Basics and Beyond. New York: Guilford Press.

Beck, N. C., J. C. Parker, R. G. Frank, E. A. Geden, D. R. Kay, M. Gamache, N. Shivvers, E. Smith, and S. Anderson (1988). Patients with rheumatoid arthritis at high risk for noncompliance with salicylate treatment regimens. *Journal of Rheumatology* 15(7):1081–1084.

Beecher, H. K. (1956). Relationship of significance of wound to pain experiences. *Journal of the American Medical Association* 161:1609–1613.

Berkman, L. F., L. Leo-Summers, and R. I. Horwitz (1992). Emotional support and survival after myocardial infarction. A prospective, population-based study of the elderly. *Annals of Internal Medicine* 117(12):1003–1009.

Berkman, L. F., and S. L. Syme (1979). Social networks, host resistance, and mortality: A nine-year follow-up study of Alameda County residents. *American Journal of Epidemiology* 109(2):186–204.

Bloom, J. R. (1982). Social support, accommodation to stress and adjustment to breast cancer. *Social Science and Medicine* 16(14):1329–1338.

Bloom, J. R., P. Fobair, and D. Spiegel (1991). Social supports and the social well-being of cancer survivors. *Advances in Medical Sociology* 2:95–114.

Bloom, J. R., and D. Spiegel (1984). The relationship of two dimensions of social support to the psychological well-being and social functioning of women with advanced breast cancer. *Social Science and Medicine* 19(8):831–837.

Bonica, J. J. (1979). Importance of the problem. *Advances in Pain Research and Therapy* 2:1–12.

Bonica, J. J. (1990). Evolution and current status of pain. *Journal of Pain Symptom Management* 5:368–374.

Borghede, G., and M. Sullivan (1996). Measurement of quality of life in localized prostatic cancer patients treated with radiotherapy. Development of a prostate cancer-specific module supplementing the EORTC QLQ-C30. *Quality of Life Research* 5(2):212–222.

Bremner, J. D., S. Southwick, E. Brett, A. Fontana, R. Rosenbeck, and D. S. Charney (1992). Dissociation and posttraumatic stress disorder in Vietnam combat veterans. *American Journal of Psychiatry* 149(3):328–332.

Brose, W. G., and D. Spiegel (1992). Neuropsychiatric aspects of pain management. In *The American Psychiatric Press Textbook of Neuropsychiatry*, S. C. Yudofsky and R. E. Hales (eds.). Washington, DC: American Psychiatric Press, Inc., pp. 245–275.

Browne, G. B., K. Arpin, P. Corey, M. Fitch, and A. Gafni (1990). Individual correlates of health service utilization and the cost of poor adjustment to chronic illness. *Medical Care* 28(1):43–58.

Bugental, J. F. (1973–1974). Confronting the existential meaning of "my death" through group exercises. *Interpersonal Development* 4(3):148–163.

Butler, L. D., C. Koopman, C. Classen, and D. Spiegel (in press). Traumatic stress, life events, and emotional support in women with metastatic breast cancer: Cancer-related traumatic stress symptoms associated with past and current stressors. *Health Psychology*.

Cacioppo, J. T. (1994). Social neuroscience: Autonomic, neuroendocrine, and immune responses to stress. *Psychophysiology* 31(2):113–128.

Cain, E. N., E. I. Kohorn, D. M. Quinlan, K. Latimer, and P. E. Schwartz (1986). Psychosocial benefits of a cancer support group. *Cancer* 57(1):183–189.

Caplan, G. (1964). *Principles of Preventive Psychiatry*. New York: Basic Books.

Cardeña, E., and D. Spiegel (1993). Dissociative reactions to the San Francisco Bay Area earthquake of 1989. *American Journal of Psychiatry* 150(3):474–478.

Cella, D. F., A. Pratt, and J. C. Holland (1986). Persistent anticipatory nausea, vomiting, and anxiety in cured Hodgkin's disease patients after completion of chemotherapy. *American Journal of Psychiatry* 143(5):641–643.

Chaves, J. F. (1994). Recent advances in the application of hypnosis to pain management. *American Journal of Clinical Hypnosis* 37(2):117–129.

Chochinov, H. M., K. G. Wilson, M. Enns, N. Mowchun, S. Lander, M. Levitt, and J. J. Clinch (1995). Desire for death in the terminally ill. *American Journal of Psychiatry* 152(8):1185–1191.

Classen, Koopman, et al. (1996). Coping styles associated with psychological adjustment to advanced breat cancer. *Health Psychology* 15(6):434–437.

Classen, C., S. Abramson, K. Angell, A. Atkinson, A. Desch, C. Vinciguerra, Rosenbluth, J. J. Kirshner, R. Hart, G. Morrow, D. Spiegel (1997). Effectiveness of a training program for enhancing therapists' understanding of the supportive-expressive treatment model for breast cancer groups. *The Journal of Psychotherapy Practice and Research*, 6(3): 211–218.

Classen, C., L. D. Butler, C. Koopman, E. Miller, S. DiMiceli, J. Giese-Davis, R. W. Carlson, H. C. Kraemer, and D. Spiegel (in submission). Supportive-expressive group therapy reduces distress in metastatic breast cancer patients: A randomized clinical intervention trial.

Classen, C., S. Diamond, and D. Spiegel, (1994). *Brief supportive-expressive group therapy for high risk breast cancer patients.* Stanford, CA: Psychosocial Treatment Laboratory, Department of Psychiatry and Behavioral Sciences, Stanford University School of Medicine.

Classen, C., C. Koopman, A. Atkinson, S. DiMiceli, G. Stonisch-Riggs, J. Westendorp, G. Morrow, and D. Spiegel (in submission). Group therapy for primary breast cancer patients: A randomized, prospective, multicenter trial.

Cohen, S., D. A. Tyrrell, and A. P. Smith (1991). Psychological stress and susceptibility to the common cold. *New England Journal of Medicine* 325(9):606–612.

Collison, D. R. (1975). Which asthmatic patients should be treated by hypnotherapy? *Medical Journal of Australia* 1(25):776–781.

Covino, N. A., and F. H. Frankel (1993). Hypnosis and relaxation in the medically ill. *Psychotherapy and Psychosomatics* 60(2):75–90.

Craig, T. J., and M. D. Abeloff (1974). Psychiatric symptomatology among hospitalized cancer patients. *American Journal of Psychiatry* 131(12):1323–1327.

Craig, T. J., G. W. Comstock, and P. B. Gieser (1974). Epidemiologic comparison of breast cancer patients with early and late onset of malignancy and general population controls. *Journal of the National Cancer Institute* 53(6):1577–1581.

Cummings, N. A., and G. R. VandenBos (1981). The twenty years Kaiser-Permanente experience with psychotherapy and medical utilization: Implications for national health policy and national health insurance. *Health Policy Q* 1(2):159–175.

Cunningham, A. J., C. V. I. Edmonds, G. P. Jenkins, H. Pollack, G. A. Lockwood, and D. Warr (1998). A randomized controlled trial of the effects of group psychological therapy on survival in women with metastatic breast cancer. *Psycho-Oncology* 7:508–517.

Dakof, G. A., and S. E. Taylor (1990). Victims' perceptions of social support: What is helpful from whom? *Journal of Personality and Social Psychology* 58(1):80–89.

da Silva, F. C. (1993). Quality of life in prostatic carcinoma. *European Urology* 24(suppl. 2):113–117.

DeAntoni, E. P., and E. D. Crawford (1994). Pretreatment of metastatic disease. Prostate cancer in the older male. *Cancer* 74(suppl. 7):2182–2187.

Derogatis, L. R., M. D. Abeloff, N. Melisaratos (1979). Psychological coping mechanisms and survival time in metastatic breast cancer. *Journal of the American Medical Association* 242(14):1504–1508.

Derogatis, L. R., G. R. Morrow, J. Fetting, D. Penman, S. Piasetsky, A. M. Schmale, M. Heinrichs, and C. L. Carnicke, Jr. (1983). The prevalence of psychiatric disorders among cancer patients. *Journal of the American Medical Association* 249(6):751–757.

Devine, E. C. (1992). Effects of psychoeducational care for adult surgical patients: A meta-analysis of 191 studies. *Patient Education and Counseling* 19(2):129–142.

DuHamel, K. N., W. H. Redd, M. Y. Smith, S. M. J. Vickberg, E. Papadapoulous, and P. Ricketts (1996). *Prevalence and Correlates of PTSD Symptoms in Breast Cancer Survivors*. Third World Congress on Psycho-Oncology, New York.

Dunkel-Schetter, C., L. G. Feinstein, S. E. Taylor, and R. L. Falke (1992). Patterns of coping with cancer. *Health Psychology* 11(2):79–87.

Edgar, L., Z. Rosberger, and D. Nowlis (1992). Coping with cancer during the first year after diagnosis. *Cancer* 69(3):817–828.

Eisenthal, S., R. Emery, A. Lazare, and H. Udin (1979). "Adherence" and the negotiated approach to patienthood. *Archives of General Psychiatry* 36(4):393–398.

Elkin, I., M. T. Shea, J. T. Watkins, S. D. Imber, S. M. Sotsky, J. F. Collins, D. R. Glass, P. A. Pilkonis, W. R. Leber, J. P. Docherty, et al. (1989). National Institute of Mental Health Treatment of Depression Collaborative Research Program. General effectiveness of treatments [see comments]. *Archives of General Psychiatry* 46(11):971–982; discussion 983.

Ell, K., R. Nishimoto, L. Mediansky, J. Mantell, and M. Hamovitch (1992). Social relations, social support and survival among patients with cancer. *Journal of Psychosomatic Research* 36(6):531–541.

Ell, K., R. Nishimoto, T. Morvay, J. Mantell, and M. Hamovitch (1989). A longitudinal analysis of psychological adaptation among survivors of cancer. *Cancer* 63(2):406–413.

Ewer, T. C., and D. E. Stewart (1986). Improvement in bronchial hyper-responsiveness in patients with moderate asthma after treatment with a hypnotic technique: A randomised controlled trial. *British Medical Journal* 293(6555):1129–1132.

Ewin, D. M. (1992). Hypnotherapy for warts (verruca vulgaris): 41 consecutive cases with 33 cures. *American Journal of Clinical Hypnosis* 35(1):1–10.

Faller, H., S. Schilling, M. Otteni, and H. Lang (1995). Social support and social stress in tumor patients and their partners. *Zeitschrift für Psychosomatische Medizin und Psychoanalyse* 41(2):141–157.

Fallowfield, L., M. Baum, and G. Macquire (1987). Effects of breast conservation on psychological morbidity associated with diagnosis and treatment of early breast cancer. *British Medical Journal* 239:1331–1334.

Fallowfield, L. J., and A. Hall (1991). Psychosocial and sexual impact of diagnosis and treatment of breast cancer. *British Medical Bulletin* 47(2):388–399.

Fawzy, F. (1991). *Effects of group support on malignant melanoma patients.* Paper presented at the Memorial Sloan-Kettering Conference on Psychosocial Oncology, New York. October.

Fawzy, F. I., N. Cousins, N. W. Fawzy, M. E. Kemeny, R. Elashoff, and D. Morton (1990). A structured psychiatric intervention for cancer patients. I. Changes over time in methods of coping and affective disturbance. *Archives of General Psychiatry* **47**(8):720–725.

Fawzy, F. I., N. W. Fawzy, L. A. Arndt, and R. O. Pasnau (1995). Critical review of psychosocial interventions in cancer care. *Archives of General Psychiatry* **52**(2):100–113.

Fawzy, F. I., N. W. Fawzy, C. Hyun, R. Elashoff, D. Guthrie, J. L. Fahey, and D. L. Morton (1993). Malignant melanoma. Effects of an early structured psychiatric intervention, coping, and affective state on recurrence and survival 6 years later. *Archives of General Psychiatry* **50**(9):681–689.

Fawzy, F. I., M. E. Kemeny, N. W. Fawzy, R. Elashoff, D. Morton, N. Cousins, and J. L. Fahey (1990). A structured psychiatric intervention for cancer patients. II. Changes over time in immunological measures. *Archives of General Psychiatry* **47**(8):729–735.

Felton, B. J., T. A. Revenson, and G. A. Hinrichsen (1984). Stress and coping in the explanation of psychological adjustment among chronically ill adults. *Social Science and Medicine* **18**(10):889–898.

Ferguson, K., and G. G. Bole (1979). Family support, health beliefs, and therapeutic compliance in patients with rheumatoid arthritis. *Patient Counseling and Health Education* **1**(3):101–105.

Ferlic, M., A. Goldman, and B. J. Kennedy (1979). Group counseling in adult patients with advanced cancer. *Cancer* **43**(2):760–766.

Fobair, P., R. T. Hoppe, J. Bloom, R. Cox, A. Varghese, and D. Spiegel (1986). Psychosocial problems among survivors of Hodgkin's disease. *Journal of Clinical Oncology* **4**(5):805–814.

Folkman, S., and R. Lazarus (1980). An analysis of coping in a middle-aged community sample. *Journal of Health and Social Behavior* **21**(3):219–239.

Forester, B., D. S. Kornfeld, and J. L. Fleiss (1985). Psychotherapy during radiotherapy: effects on emotional and physical distress. *American Journal of Psychiatry* **142**(1):22–27.

Frankel, F. H. (1987). Significant developments in medical hypnosis during the past 25 years. *International Journal of Clinical and Experimental Hypnosis* **35**(4):231–247.

Friedman, L. C., P. E. Baer, D. V. Nelson, M. Lane, F. E. Smith, and R. J. Dworkin (1988). Women with breast cancer: perception of family functioning and adjustment to illness. *Psychosomatic Medicine* **50**(5):529–540.

Front, D., S. O. Schneck, et al. (1979). Bone metastases and bone pain in breast cancer: Are they associated? *Journal of the American Medical Association* **242**:1747–1748.

Funch, D. P., and J. Marshall (1983). The role of stress, social support and age in survival from breast cancer. *Journal of Psychosomatic Research* **27**(1):77–83.

Ganster, D. C., and B. Victor (1988). The impact of social support on mental and physical health. *British Journal of Medical Psychology* **61**(Pt 1):17–36.

Ganz, P. A., J. J. Lee, M. S. Sim, M. L. Polinsky, and C. A. Schag (1992). Exploring the influence of multiple variables on the relationship of age to quality of life in women with breast cancer. *Journal of Clinical Epidemiology* **45**(5):473–485.

Garfinkel, M. S., A. Singhal, W. A. Katz, D. A. Allen, R. Reshetar, and H. R. Schumacher (1998). Yoga-based intervention for carpal tunnel syndrome: A randomized trial. *Journal of the American Medical Association* **280**(18):1601–1603.

Gellert, G. A., R. M. Maxwell, and B. S. Siegel (1993). Survival of breast cancer patients receiving adjunctive psychosocial support therapy: a 10-year follow-up study. *Journal of Clinical Oncology* **11**(1):66–69.

Geyer, S. (1991). Life events prior to manifestation of breast cancer: a limited prospective study covering eight years before diagnosis. *Journal of Psychosomatic Research* **35**(2–3):355–363.

Given, B. A., and C. W. Given (1989). Compliance among patients with cancer. *Oncology Nursing Forum* **16**(1):97–103.

Glaser, R., and J. K. Kiecolt-Glaser (1986). Stress and immune function. *Clinical Neuropharmacology* **9 Suppl 4**:485–487.

Glaser, R., J. K. Kiecolt-Glaser, W. B. Malarkes, and J. F. Sheridan (1998). The influence of psychological stress on the immune response to vaccines. *Annals of the New York Academy of Sciences* **840**:649–655.

Glaser, R., J. K. Kiecolt-Glaser, J. C. Stout, K. L. Tarr, C. E. Speicher, and J. E. Holliday (1985). Stress-related impairments in cellular immunity. *Psychiatry Research* **16**(3):233–239.

Glass, A., H. S. Wieand, B. Fisher, C. Redmond, H. Lerner, J. Wolter, H. Shibata, D. Plotkin, R. Foster, R. Margolese, and N. Wolmark (1981). Acute toxicity during adjuvant chemotherapy for breast cancer: The National Surgical Adjuvant Breast and Bowel Project (NSABP) experience from 1,717 patients receiving single and multiple agents. *Cancer Treatment Reports* **65**(5–6):363–376.

Goodwin, J. S., W. C. Hunt, C. R. Key, and J. M. Samet (1987). The effect of marital status on stage, treatment, and survival of cancer patients. *Journal of the American Medical Association* **258**(21):3125–3130.

Goodwin, P. J., M. Leszcz, et al. (1996). Randomized trial of group psychosocial support in metastatic breast cancer: The BEST (Breast Expressive-Supportive Therapy) study. *Cancer Treatment Reviews* **22**(suppl. A):91–96.

Greer, S. (1991). Psychological response to cancer and survival. *Psychological Medicine* **21**(1):43–49.

Greer, S. (1993). Psycho-oncology: Its aims, achievements and future tasks. *Psycho-Oncology* **3**:87–102.

Greer, S., and T. Morris (1975). Psychological attributes of women who develop breast cancer: a controlled study. *Journal of Psychosomatic Research* **19**(2):147–153.

Greer, S., T. Morris, and K. W. Pettingale (1979). Psychological response to breast cancer: effect on outcome. *Lancet* **2**(8146):785–787.

Gritz, E. R., D. K. Wellisch, J. Siau, and H. J. Wang (1990). Long-term effects of testicular cancer on marital relationships. *Psychosomatics* **31**(3):301–312.

Gustafson, J., and H. Whitman (1978). Towards a balanced social environment on the oncology service. *Social Psychiatry* **13**:147–152.

Hannah, M. T., E. R. Gritz, D. K. Wellisch, P. Fobair, R. T. Hoppe, J. R. Bloom, G. W. Sun, A. Varghese, M. D. Cosgrove, and D. Spiegel (1992). Changes in marital and sexual functioning in long-term survivors and their spouses: Testicular cancer versus Hodgkin's disease. *Psycho-Oncology* 1:89–103.

Harris, J. R., M. E. Lippman, U. Veronesi, and W. Willett (1992). Breast cancer. *New England Journal of Medicine* (review articles) 327(6):390–398.

Hastorf, A. H., J. Wildfogel, and T. Cassman (1979). Acknowledgment of handicap as a tactic in social interaction. *Journal of Personality and Social Psychology* 37(10):1790–1797.

Havlik, R. J., A. P. Vukasin, and S. Ariyan (1992). The impact of stress on the clinical presentation of melanoma. *Plastic and Reconstructive Surgery* 90(1):57–61; discussion 62–64.

Haynes, B., D. Taylor, et al., eds. (1979). *Compliance in Health Care.* Baltimore: Johns Hopkins University Press.

Helgeson, V., S. Cohen, R. Schulz, and J. Yasko (1999). Education and peer discussion group interventions and adjustment to breast cancer. *Archives of General Psychiatry* 56(4):340–347.

Hellman, C. J., M. Budd, J. Borysenko, D. C. McClelland, and H. Benson (1990). A study of the effectiveness of two group behavioral medicine interventions for patients with psychosomatic complaints. *Behavioral Medicine* 16(4):165–173.

Henderson, I. C., J. E. Garber, J. B. Breitmeyer, D. F. Hayes, and J. R. Harris (1990). Comprehensive management of disseminated breast cancer. *Cancer* 66(6 Suppl):1439–1448.

Hendler, N. (1984). Depression caused by chronic pain. *Journal of Clinical Psychiatry* 45(3, part 2):30–38.

Hilgard, E. (1965). *Hypnotic Susceptibility.* New York: Harcourt, Brace & World.

Hilgard, E. R. (1991). Suggestibility and suggestions as related to hypnosis. In *Human Suggestibility: Advances in Theory, Research, and Application,* J. F. Schumaker (ed.). New York: Routledge, pp. 37–58.

Hilgard, E. R., and J. R. Hilgard (1975). *Hypnosis in the Relief of Pain.* Los Altos: William Kauffman.

Hilgard, J. R., and S. LeBaron (1982). Relief of anxiety and pain in children and adolescents with cancer: Quantitative measures and clinical observations. *International Journal of Clinical and Experimental Hypnosis* 4:417–442.

Hislop, T. G., N. E. Waxler, A. J. Coldman, J. M. Elwood, and L. Kan (1987). The prognostic significance of psychosocial factors in women with breast cancer. *Journal of Chronic Diseases* 40(7):729–735.

Hoagland, A. C., G. R. Morrow, J. M. Bennett, and C. Carnrike, Jr. (1983). Oncologists' views of cancer patient noncompliance. *American Journal of Clinical Oncology* 6(2):239–244.

Hobson, J. A., and R. Stickgold (1995). Sleep. Sleep the beloved teacher? *Current Biology* 5(1):35–36.

Holland, J., and R. J. Holland, eds. (1989). *Handbook of Psychooncology: Psychologic Care of the Patient with Cancer.* Newark: Oxford University Press.

Holroyd, J. (1996). Hypnosis treatment of clinical pain: Understanding why hypnosis is useful. *International Journal of Clinical and Experimental Hypnosis* 44(1):33–51.

House, J. S., K. R. Landis, and D. Umberson (1988). Social relationships and health. *Science* 241(4865):540–545.

House, J. S., J. M. Lepkowski, A. M. Kenney, R. P. Mero, R. C. Kessler, and A. Herzog (1994). The social stratification of aging and health. *Journal of Health and Social Behavior* 35(3):213–234.

House, J. S., C. Robbins, and H. L. Metzner (1982). The association of social relationships and activities with mortality: prospective evidence from the Tecumseh Community Health Study. *American Journal of Epidemiology* 116(1):123–140.

Hughes, J. (1982). Emotional reactions to the diagnosis and treatment of early breast cancer. *Journal of Psychosomatic Research* 26(2):277–283.

Hughes, J. E., G. T. Royle, R. Buchanan, and J. Taylor (1986). Depression and social stress among patients with benign breast disease. *British Journal of Surgery* 73(12):997–999.

Ilnyckyj, A., J. Farber, M. Cheang, and B. Weinerman (1994). A randomized controlled trial of psychotherapeutic intervention in cancer patients. *Annals of the Royal College of Physicians and Surgeons of Canada* 27(2):93–96.

Irvine, D., B. Brown, D. Crooks, J. Roberts, and G. Browne (1991). Psychosocial adjustment in women with breast cancer. *Cancer* 67(4):1097–1117.

Itano, J. K., P. H. Tanabe, J. Lum, L. Lamkin, E. Rizzo, M. Wieland, and P. Sato (1983a). Compliance and noncompliance in cancer patients. *Progress in Clinical and Biological Research* 120:483–495.

Itano, J., P. Tanabe, J. L. Lum, L. Lamkin, E. Rizzo, M. Wieland, and P. Sato (1983b). Compliance of cancer patients to therapy. *Western Journal of Nursing Research* 5(1):5–20.

Jamison, K. R., D. K. Wellisch, and R. O. Pasnau (1978). Psychosocial aspects of mastectomy: I. The women's perspective. *American Journal of Psychiatry* 135(4):432–436.

Joffres , M., D. M. Reed, and A. M. Nomura (1985). Psychosocial processes and cancer incidence among Japanese men in Hawaii. *American Journal of Epidemiology* 121(4):488–500.

Kabat-Zinn, J. (1994). *Full Catastophe Living: Using the Wisdom of Your Body and Mind to Face Stress, Pain and Illness.* New York: Delacorte Press.

Katon, W., and M. Sullivan (1990). Depression and chronic medical illness. *Journal of Behavioral Medicine* 11:3–11.

Katz, R. L., C. Y. Kao, H. Spiegel, and G. J. Katz (1974). Acupuncture and hypnosis. *Advances in Neurology* 4:819–825.

Kaye, J. M., and E. J. Gracely (1993). Psychological distress in cancer patients and their spouses. *Journal of Cancer Education* 8(1):47–52.

Kelly, J. A., D. A. Murphy, G. R. Bahr, S. C. Kalichman, M. G. Morgan, L. Y. Stevenson, J. J. Koob, T. L. Brasfield, and B. M. Bernstein (1993). Outcome of cognitive-behavioral and support group brief therapies for depressed HIV-infected persons. *American Journal of Psychiatry* 150(11):1679–1686.

Kennedy, S., J. K. Kiecolt-Glaser, and R. Glaser (1988). Immunological consequences of acute and chronic stressors: Mediating role of interpersonal relationships. *British Journal of Medical Psychology* 61(Pt 1):77–85.

Kierkegaard, S. (1843; 1848; reprint 1954). *Fear and Trembling and the Sickness Unto Death*, W. Lowrie, trans. Garden City, NY: Doubleday.

Knox, V. J., and K. Shum (1977). Reduction of cold-pressor pain with acupuncture analgesia in high- and low-hypnotic subjects. *Journal of Abnormal Psychology* 86(6):639–643.

Kogon, M., A. Biswas, D. Pearl, R. Carlson, and D. Spiegel (1997). Effects of medical and psychotherapeutic treatment on the survival of women with metastatic breast carcinoma. *Cancer* 80(2):225–230.

Kohen, D. P., K. N. Olness, S. O. Colwell, and A. Heimel (1984). The use of relaxation-mental imagery (self-hypnosis) in the management of 505 pediatric behavioral encounters. *Journal of Developmental and Behavioral Pediatrics* 5(1):21–25.

Koocher, G., and J. O'Malley (1981). *The Damocles Syndrome: Psychosocial Consequences of Surviving Childhood Cancer*. New York: McGraw-Hill.

Koopman, C., C. Classen, and D. Spiegel (1994). Predictors of posttraumatic stress symptoms among survivors of the Oakland/Berkeley, Calif., firestorm. *American Journal of Psychiatry* 151(6):888–894.

Krupnick, J. (1996). Life-threatening illness and posttraumatic stress disorder (PTSD). In *Psychosocial responses to breast cancer*. Psychosocial and Behavioral Factors in Women's Health: Research, prevention, treatment and service delivery in clinical and community settings, Washington, D.C.

Krupnick, J., J. Rowland, R. Goldberg, and U. Daniel (1993). Professionally-led support groups for cancer patients: an intervention in search of a model. *Psychiatry in Medicine* 23(3):275–294.

Kupst, M. J. (1993). Family coping. Supportive and obstructive factors. *Cancer* 71(suppl. 10):3337–3341.

Lambert, S. A. (1996). The effects of hypnosis/guided imagery on the postoperative course of children. *Journal of Developmental and Behavioral Pediatrics* 17(5):307–310.

Lang, E., J. Joyce, D. Spiegel, D. Hamilton, and K. Lee (1996). Self-hypnotic relaxation during interventional radiological procedures: Effects on pain perception and intravenous drug use. *International Journal of Clinical and Experimental Hypnosis* XLIV(2):106–119.

Lansky, S. B., M. A. List, C. A. Herrmann, E. G. Ets-Hokin, T. K. DasGupta, G. D. Wilbanks, and J. R. Hendrickson (1985). Absence of major depressive disorder in female cancer patients. *Journal of Clinical Oncology* 3(11):1553–1560.

Laszlo, J., and V. Lucas, Jr. (1981). Emesis as a critical problem in chemotherapy [editorial]. *New England Journal of Medicine* 305(16):948–949.

Lee, Y. T. (1983). Adjuvant chemotherapy (CMF) for breast carcinoma. Patient's compliance and total dose achieved. *American Journal of Clinical Oncology* 6(1):25–30.

Lerman, C., E. Lustbader, B. Rimer, M. Daly, S. Miller, C. Sands, and A. Balshman (1995). Effects of individualized breast cancer risk counseling: a randomized trial. *Journal of the National Cancer Institute* 87:286–292.

Levine, S., C. Coe, and S. G. Wiener (1989). Psychoneuroendocrinology of stress: a psychobiological perspective. In *Psychoendocrinology*. F. R. Brush and S. Levine, eds. New York: Academic Press.

Levy, S., R. Herberman, J. Lee, M. Lippman, and R. d'Angelo (1989). Breast conservation versus mastectomy: Distress sequelae as a function of choice. *Journal of Clinical Oncology* 7:367–375.

Lewis, F. M., and M. A. Hammond (1992). Psychosocial adjustment of the family to breast cancer: a longitudinal analysis. *Journal of the American Medical Women's Association* 47(5):194–200.

Liang, L. P., S. M. Dunn, A. Gorman, and R. Stuart-Harris (1990). Identifying priorities of psychosocial need in cancer patients. *British Journal of Cancer* 62(6):1000–1003.

Lindemann, E. (1994; first published in 1944). Symptomatology and management of acute grief. *American Journal of Psychiatry* 151(6 Suppl):155–160.

Linn, M. W., B. S. Linn, and R. Harris (1982). Effects of counseling for late stage cancer. *Cancer* 49:1048–1055.

Lipsey, M. W., and D. B. Wilson (1993). The efficacy of psychological, educational, and behavioral treatment: Confirmation from meta-analysis. *American Psychologist* 48(12):1181–1209.

Lorig, K., D. Lubeck, R. G. Kraines, M. Seleznick, and H. R. Holman (1985). Outcomes of self-help education for patients with arthritis. *Arthritis and Rheumatism* 28(6):680–685.

Lyles, J. N., T. G. Burish, M. G. Krozely, and R. K. Oldham (1982). Efficacy of relaxation training and guided imagery in reducing the aversiveness of cancer chemotherapy. *Journal of Consulting and Clinical Psychology* 50(4):509–524.

Maguire, G. P., E. G. Lee, D. J. Bevington, C. S. Kuchemann, R. J. Crabtree, and E. C. Cornell (1978). Psychiatric problems in the first year after mastectomy. *British Medical Journal* 1(6118):963–965.

Mahon, S. M., D. F. Cella, and M. I. Donovan (1990). Psychosocial adjustment to recurrent cancer. *Oncology Nursing Forum* 17(3 Suppl):47–52; discussion 53–54.

Maldonado, J., and D. Spiegel, eds. (1996). *Hypnosis. Psychiatry*. Philadelphia: W. B. Saunders.

Maldonado, J. R., and D. Spiegel (1998). Trauma, dissociation and hypnotizability. In *Trauma, Memory and Dissociation*, R. Marmar and D. Bremmer (eds.). Washington, DC: American Psychiatric Press.

Maraste, R., L. Brandt, H. Olsson, and B. Ryde-Brandt (1992). Anxiety and depression in breast cancer patients at start of adjuvant radiotherapy. Relations to age and type of surgery. *Acta Oncologica* 31(6):641–643.

Marcus, A. C., L. A. Crane, C. P. Kaplan, A. E. Reading, E. Savage, J. Gunning, G. Bernstein, and J. S. Berek (1992). Improving adherence to screening follow-up among women with abnormal Pap smears: results from a large clinic-based trial of three intervention strategies. *Medical Care* 30(3):216–230.

Marmar, C. R., D. S. Weiss, W. E. Schlenger, J. A. Fairbank, B. K. Jordan, R. A. Kulka, and R. L. Hough (1994). Peritraumatic dissociation and posttraumatic stress in male Vietnam theater veterans. *American Journal of Psychiatry* 151(6):902–907.

Maslach, C., G. Marshall, and P. G. Zimbardo (1972). Hypnotic control of peripheral skin temperature: A case report. *Psychophysiology* 9(6):600–605.

Massie, M. J., and J. C. Holland (1987). The cancer patient with pain: psychiatric complications and their management. *Medical Clinics of North America* 71(2):243–258.

Massie, M. J., and J. C. Holland (1990). Depression and the cancer patient. *Journal of Clinical Psychiatry* 51:12–17; discussion 18–19.

Maunsell, E., J. Brisson, and L. Deschenes (1992). Psychological distress after initial treatment of breast cancer. Assessment of potential risk factors. *Cancer* 70(1):120–125.

Maunsell, E., B. Jacques, and L. Deschenes (1995). Social support and survival among women with breast cancer. *Cancer* 76(4):631–637.

McDaniel, J. S., D. L. Musselman, M. R. Porter, D. A. Reed, and C. B. Nemeroff (1995). Depression in patients with cancer. Diagnosis, biology, and treatment. *Archives of General Psychiatry* 52(2):89–99.

McDaniel, J. S., and C. B. Nemeroff (1993). Depression in the cancer patient: diagnostic, biological, and treatment aspects. In *Current and Emerging Issues in Cancer Pain: Research and Practice*. C. R. Chapman and K. M. Foley. New York: Raven Press, pp. 1–19.

McEwen, B. S. (1998). Protective and damaging effects of stress mediators. *New England Journal of Medicine* 338(3):171–179.

McFarlane, A. C. (1986). Posttraumatic morbidity of a disaster. A study of cases presenting for psychiatric treatment. *Journal of Nervous and Mental Disease* 174(1):4–14.

McNair, D. M., M. Lorr, and L. F. Droppleman (1992). Edits Manual for the Profile of Mood States, Educational and Industrial Testing Service.

Mermelstein, H. T., and L. Lesko (1992). Depression in patients with cancer. *Psychooncology* 1:199–225.

Moore, M. E., and S. N. Berk (1976). Acupuncture for chronic shoulder pain. An experimental study with attention to the role of placebo and hypnotic susceptibility. *Annals of Internal Medicine* 84(4):381–384.

Moos, R. H., and J. A. Schaefer (1987). The crisis of physical illness: An overview and conceptual approach. In *Coping with Physical Illness 2: New Perspectives*. R. H. Moos. New York: Plenum.

Morgenstern, H., G. A. Gellert, S. D. Walter, A. M. Ostfeld, and B. S. Siegel (1984). The impact of a psychosocial support program on survival with breast cancer: the importance of selection bias in program evaluation. *Journal of Chronic Diseases* 37(4):273–282.

Morris, T., and S. Greer (1982). Psychological characteristics of women electing to attend a breast screening clinic. *Clinical Oncology* 8(2):113–119.

Morris, T., H. S. Greer, and P. White (1977). Psychological and social adjustment to mastectomy: a two-year follow-up study. *Cancer* 40(5):2381–2387.

Morrison, J. B. (1988). Chronic asthma and improvement with relaxation induced by hypnotherapy [see comments]. *Journal of the Royal Society of Medicine* 81(12):701–704.

Morrow, G. R., and C. Morrell (1982). Behavioral treatment for the anticipatory nausea and vomiting induced by cancer chemotherapy. *New England Journal of Medicine* 307(24):1476–1480.

Motzer, R. J., N. L. Geller, and G. L. Bosl (1990). The effect of a 7-day delay in chemotherapy cycles on complete response and event-free survival in good-risk disseminated germ cell tumor patients. *Cancer* 66(5):857–861.

Mulder, C., G. van der Pompe, D. Spiegel, and M. Antoni (1992). Do psychosocial factors influence the course of breast cancer? A review of recent literature methodological problems and future directions. *Psycho-oncology* 1:155–167.

Mumford, E., H. J. Schlesinger, G. V. Glass, C. Patrick, and T. Cuerdon (1984). A new look at evidence about reduced cost of medical utilization following mental health treatment. *American Journal of Psychiatry* 141(10):1145–1158.

Myers, J. K., M. M. Weissman, G. L. Tischler, C. D. Holzer, P. J. Leaf, H. Orvaschel, J. C. Anthony, J. H. Boyd, J. Burke, Jr., M. Kramer, et al. (1984). Six-month prevalence of psychiatric disorders in three communities 1980 to 1982. *Archives of General Psychiatry* 41(10):959–967.

Northouse, L. L. (1981). Mastectomy patients and the fear of cancer recurrence. *Cancer Nursing* 4(3):213–220.

Northouse, L. L. (1989). The impact of breast cancer on patients and husbands. *Cancer Nursing* 12(5):276–284.

Northouse, L. L., and M. A. Swain (1987). Adjustment of patients and husbands to the initial impact of breast cancer. *Nursing Research* 36(4):221–225.

Omne-Ponten, M., L. Holmberg, T. Burns, H. O. Adami, and R. Bergstrom (1992). Determinants of the psycho-social outcome after operation for breast cancer. Results of a prospective comparative interview study following mastectomy and breast conservation. *European Journal of Cancer* 28A(6–7):1062–1067.

Omne-Ponten, M., L. Holmberg, and P. O. Sjoden (1994). Psychosocial adjustment among women with breast cancer stages I and II: six-year follow-up of consecutive patients. *Journal of Clinical Oncology* 12(9):1778–1782.

Patterson, D. R., J. J. Everett, G. L. Burns, and J. A. Marvin (1992). Hypnosis for the treatment of burn pain. *Journal of Consulting and Clinical Psychology* 60(5):713–717.

Pelletier, K. R., A. Marie, M. Krasner, and W. L. Haskell (1997). Current Trends in the Integration and Reimbursement of Complementary and Alternative Medicine by Managed Care, Insurance Carriers, and Hospital Providers. *American Journal of Health Promotion* 12(2):112–122.

Primomo, J., B. C. Yates, and N. F. Woods (1990). Social support for women during chronic illness: The relationship among sources and types to adjustment. *Research in Nursing and Health* 13(3):153–161.

Public Health Service (1993). *Depression in Primary Care: Vol. 2. Treatment of major depression.* Rockville, MD: Public Health Service, Agency for Health Care Policy and Research.

Quigley, K. M. (1989). The adult cancer survivor: psychosocial consequences of cure. *Seminars in Oncology Nursing* 5(1):63–69.

Ramirez, A. J., T. K. Craig, J. P. Watson, I. S. Fentiman, W. R. North, and R. D. Rubens (1989). Stress and relapse of breast cancer [see comments]. *British Medical Journal* 298(6669):291–293.

Raphael, B. (1977). Preventive intervention with the recently bereaved. *Archives of General Psychiatry* 34(12):1450–1454.

Reynolds, P., and G. A. Kaplan (1990). Social connections and risk for cancer: prospective evidence from the Alameda County Study. *Behavioral Medicine* 16(3):101–110.

Richardson, J. L., D. R. Shelton, M. Krailo, and A. M. Levine (1990). The effect of compliance with treatment on survival among patients with hematologic malignancies. *Journal of Clinical Oncology* 8(2):356–364.

Richmond, K., B. M. Berman, J. P. Docherty, L. B. Holdstein, G. Kaplan, J. E. Keil, S. Krippner, S. Lyne, F. Mosteller, B. B. O'Connor, E. B. Rudy, and A. F. Schatzberg (1996). Integration of behavioral and relaxation approaches into the treatment of chronic pain and insomnia. *Journal of the American Medical Association* 276:313–318.

Rieker, P. P., S. D. Edbril, and M. B. Garnick (1985). Curative testis cancer therapy: psychosocial sequelae. *Journal of Clinical Oncology* 3(8):1117–1126.

Riessman, F. (1965). The "helper" therapy principle. *Social Work* 10:27–32.

Rodin, G., and K. Voshart (1986). Depression in the medically ill: an overview. *American Journal of Psychiatry* 143(6):696–705.

Rodin, J. (1980). *Managing the stress of aging: the role of control and coping.* New York: Plenum.

Rodin, J. (1986). *Health, control and aging.* Hillsdale, NJ: Earlbaum.

Rogers, C. R. (1957). The necessary and sufficient conditions of therapeutic personality change. *Journal of Consulting and Clinical Psychology* 21(2):95–103.

Rogers, C. R. (1961) *On Becoming a Person.* Boston: Houghton Mifflin Co.

Rogers, C. R. (1970). *Carl Rogers on Encounter Groups.* New York: Harper & Row.

Schottenfeld, D., and G. F. Robbins (1970). Quality of survival among patients who have had radical mastectomy. *Cancer* 26(3):650–655.

Sharp, J. W., D. Blum, and L. Aviv (1993). Elderly men with cancer: social work interventions in prostate cancer. *Social Work Health Care* 19(1):91–107.

Sinclair-Gieben, A. H. C., and D. Chalmers (1959). Evaluation of treatment of warts by hypnosis. *The Lancet* 2:480–482.

Solomon, Z., and M. Mikulincer (1988). Psychological sequelae of war. A 2-year follow-up study of Israeli combat stress reaction casualties. *Journal of Nervous and Mental Disease* 176(5):264–269.

Spanos, N. P., R. J. Stenstrom, and J. C. Johnston (1988). Hypnosis, placebo, and suggestion in the treatment of warts. *Psychosomatic Medicine* 50(3):245–260.

Spanos, N. P., V. Williams, and M. I. Gwynn (1990). Effects of hypnotic, placebo, and salicylic acid treatments on wart regression. *Psychosomatic Medicine* 52(1):109–114.

Spiegel, D. (1979). Psychological support for women with metastatic carcinoma. *Psychosomatics* 20:780–787.

Spiegel, D. (1985). The use of hypnosis in controlling cancer pain. *CA: A Cancer Journal for Clinicians* 35(4):221–231.

Spiegel, D. (1990). Facilitating emotional coping during treatment. *Cancer* 66(6 Suppl):1422–1426.

Spiegel, D. (1991). Uses of hypnosis in managing medical symptoms. *Psychiatric Medicine* 9(4):521–533.

Spiegel, D. (1993a). *Living Beyond Limits: New Help and Hope for Facing Life-Threatening Illness.* New York: Times Books/Random House.

Spiegel, D. (1993b). Psychosocial intervention in cancer. *Journal of the National Cancer Institute* 85(5):1198–1205.

Spiegel, D. (1994a). Hypnosis and Suggestion. In *Memory Distortion*. D. L. Schacter, J. T. Coyle, G. Fischback, M. M. Mesulam and L. E. Sullivan. Cambridge: Harvard University Press.

Spiegel, D. (1994b). *Living Beyond Limits*. New York: Ballantine/Fawcett.

Spiegel, D. (1997). Trauma, Dissociation, and Memory. In *Psychobiology of Posttraumatic Stress Disorder*. R. Yehuda and A. C. McFarlane. New York: The New York Academy of Sciences, pp. 225–237.

Spiegel, D., and J. R. Bloom (1983a). Group therapy and hypnosis reduce metastatic breast carcinoma pain. *Psychosomatic Medicine* 45(4):333–339.

Spiegel, D., and J. R. Bloom (1983b). Pain in metastatic breast cancer. *Cancer* 52(2):341–345.

Spiegel, D., J. R. Bloom, and E. Gottheil (1983). Family Environment as a Predictor of Adjustment to Metastatic Breast Carcinoma. *Journal of Psychosocial Oncology* 1(1):33–44.

Spiegel, D., J. R. Bloom, H. C. Kraemer, and E. Gottheil (1989). Effect of psychosocial treatment on survival of patients with metastatic breast cancer. *Lancet* 2(8668):888–891.

Spiegel, D., J. R. Bloom, and I. Yalom (1981). Group support for patients with metastatic cancer. A randomized outcome study. *Archives of General Psychiatry* 38(5):527–533.

Spiegel, D., and E. Cardeña (1991). Disintegrated experience: the dissociative disorders revisited. *Journal of Abnormal Psychology* 100(3):366–378.

Spiegel, D., and C. Classen (1995). *Acute Stress Disorder: Treatment of Psychiatric Disorders: Anxiety, Dissociative, and Adjustment Disorders*. Washington, DC: American Psychiatric Press.

Spiegel, D., and M. C. Glafkides (1983). Effects of group confrontation with death and dying. *International Journal of Group Psychotherapy* 33(4):433–447.

Spiegel, D., T. Hunt, and H. E. Dondershire (1988). Dissociation and hypnotizability in posttraumatic stress disorder. *American Journal of Psychiatry* 145(3):301–305.

Spiegel, D., and P. Kato (1996). Psychosocial influences on cancer incidence and progression. *Harvard Review of Psychiatry* 4:10–26.

Spiegel, D., and J. Maldonado (1999). Hypnosis. In *American Psychiatric Press Textbook of Psychiatry*. R. E. Hales, S. Yudofsky and J. Talbott. Washington, DC: American Psychiatric Press.

Spiegel, D., G. Morrow, C. Classen, G. Riggs, P. Stott, N. Mudalier, H. Pierce, P. Flynn, and L. Heard (1996). Effect of group therapy on women with primary breast cancer. *The Breast Journal* 2(1):104–116.

Spiegel, D., S. Sands, and C. Koopman (1994). Pain and depression in patients with cancer. *Cancer* 74(9):2570–2578.

Spiegel, D., P. Stroud, and A. Lyle (1998). Complementary Medicine. *The Western Journal of Medicine* 168:241–247.

Spiegel, D., and E. Vermetten (1993). Somatic and neurophysiological effects of hypnosis and dissociation. In *Dissociation: Culture, Mind and Body*. D. Spiegel. Washington, DC: American Psychiatric Press.

Spiegel, D., and T. Wissler (1983). Perceptions of family environment among psychiatric patients and their wives. *Family Process* 22(4):537–547.

Spiegel, D., and I. Yalom (1978). A support group for dying patients. *International Journal of Group Psychotherapy* 28:233–245.

Spiegel, H. (1974). The grade 5 syndrome: the highly hypnotizable person. *International Journal of Clinical and Experimental Hypnosis* 22(4):303–319.

Spiegel, H., and D. Spiegel (1978). *Trance and treatment: Clinical uses of hypnosis.* Washington, DC: American Psychiatric Press.

Stavraky, K. M., A. P. Donner, J. E. Kincade, and M. A. Stewart (1988). The effect of psychosocial factors on lung cancer mortality at one year. *Journal of Clinical Epidemiology* 41(1):75–82.

Steckel, S. (1982). Predicting, measuring, implementing and following up on patient compliance. *Nursing Clinics of North America* 17(3):491–498.

Strain, J. J., J. S. Lyons, J. S. Hammer, M. Lahs, A. Lebovits, P. L. Paddison, S. Snyder, E. Strauss, R. Burton, et al. (1991). Cost offset from a psychiatric consultation-liaison intervention with elderly hip fracture patients [see comments]. *American Journal of Psychiatry* 148(8):1044–1049.

Strang, P., and H. Qvarner (1990). Cancer-related pain and its influence on quality of life. *Anticancer Research* 10(1):109–112.

Study, P. A. o. B. C. (1987). Group psychological response to mastectomy: A prospective comparison study. *Cancer* 59(1):189–196.

Sullivan, H. S. (1953). *The Interpersonal Theory of Psychiatry.* New York: W. W. Norton.

Sullivan, H. S. (1954). *The Psychiatric Interview.* New York: W. W. Norton.

Surman, O. S., S. K. Gottlieb, T. P. Hackett, and E. L. Silverberg (1973). Hypnosis in the treatment of warts. *Archives of General Psychiatry* 28(3):439–441.

Taylor, S., and G. Dakof (1988). *Social support and the cancer patient.* Newbury Park, CA: Sage.

Taylor, S. E., and M. Lobel (1989). Social comparison activity under threat: downward evaluation and upward contacts. *Psychological Review* 96(4):569–575.

Telch, C. F., and M. J. Telch (1986). Group coping skills instruction and supportive group therapy for cancer patients: a comparison of strategies. *Journal of Consulting and Clinical Psychology* 54(6):802–808.

Tellegen, A., and G. Atkinson (1974). Openness to absorbing and self-altering experiences ("absorption"), a trait related to hypnotic susceptibility. *Journal of Abnormal Psychology* 83(3):268–277.

Temoshok, L. (1985). Biopsychosocial studies on cutaneous malignant melanoma: psychosocial factors associated with prognostic indicators, progression, psychophysiology and tumor-host response. *Social Science and Medicine* 20(8):833–840.

Timko, C., and R. Janoff-Bulman (1985). Attributions, vulnerability, and psychological adjustment: the case of breast cancer. *Health Psychology* 4(6):521–544.

Toseland, R. W., and L. Hacker (1982). Self-help groups and professional involvement. *Social Work* 27(4):341–347.

Tracy, G., and Z. Gussow (1976). Self-help groups: A grass-roots response to a need for services. *Journal of Applied Behavioral Science* 12:381–396.

Trijsburg, R. W., F. C. van Knippenberg, and S. E. Rijpma (1992). Effects of psychological treatment on cancer patients: a critical review. *Psychosomatic Medicine* 54(4):489–517.

Tross, S., and J. Holland (1990). Psychological sequelae in cancer survivors. In *Psychooncology: Psychological care of the patient with cancer*. J. Holland and J. Rowland. New York: Oxford University Press: 101–116.

Turner, R. J. (1981). Social support as a contingency to psychological well-being. *Journal of Health and Social Behavior* 22:357–367.

Turns, D. M. (1988). Psychosocial Factors. In W. L. Donegan and J. S. Spratt (Eds.), *Cancer of the Breast* (Third ed., pp. 728–738). Philadelphia: W. B. Saunders.

Van Cauter, E., R. Leproult, and D. J. Kupfer (1996). Effects of gender and age on the levels and circadian rhythmicity of plasma cortisol. *Journal of Clinical Endocrinology and Metabolism* 81(7):2468–2473.

Vinokur, A. D., B. A. Threatt, R. D. Caplan, and B. L. Zimmerman (1989). Physical and psychosocial functioning and adjustment to breast cancer. Long-term follow-up of a screening population. *Cancer* 63(2):394–405.

Vinokur, A. D., B. A. Threatt, D. Vinokur-Kaplan, and W. A. Satariano (1990). The process of recovery from breast cancer for younger and older patients. Changes during the first year. *Cancer* 65(5):1242–1254.

Von Korff, M., J. Ormel, W. Katon, and E. H. Lin (1992). Disability and depression among high utilizers of health care. A longitudinal analysis. *Archives of General Psychiatry* 49(2):91–100.

Watson, C. P., and R. J. Evans (1982). Intractable pain with breast cancer. *Canadian Medical Association Journal* 126(3):263–266.

Watson, M., J. Pruyn, S. Greer, and B. van den Borne (1990). Locus of control and adjustment to cancer. *Psychological Reports* 66(1):39–48.

Waxler-Morrison, N., T. G. Hislop, B. Mears, and L. Kan (1991). Effects of social relationships on survival for women with breast cancer: a prospective study. *Social Science and Medicine* 33(2):177–183.

Weisenberg, M., O. Aviram, Y. Wolf, and N. Raphaeli (1984). Relevant and irrelevant anxiety in the reaction to pain. *Pain* 20(4):371–383.

Wellisch, D., M. Mosher, and C. V. Scoy (1978). Management of family emotion stress: Family group therapy in a private oncology practice. *International Journal of Group Psychotherapy* 23:225–231.

Wells, K. B., A. Stewart, R. D. Hays, M. A. Burnam, W. Rogers, M. Daniels, S. Berry, S. Greenfield, and J. Ware (1989). The functioning and well-being of depressed patients. Results from the Medical Outcomes Study [see comments]. *Journal of the American Medical Association* 262(7):914–919.

Whorwell, P. J., A. Prior, and S. M. Colgan (1987). Hypnotherapy in severe irritable bowel syndrome: further experience. *Gut* 28:423–425.

Whorwell, P. J., A. Prior, and E. B. Faragher (1984). Controlled trial of hypnotherapy in the treatment of severe refractory irritable-bowel syndrome. *Lancet* 2(8414):1232–1234.

Wilcox, P. M., J. H. Fetting, K. M. Nettesheim, and M. D. Abeloff (1982). Anticipatory vomiting in women receiving cyclophosphamide, methotrexate, and 5-FU (CMF) adjuvant chemotherapy for breast carcinoma. *Cancer Treatment Reports* 66(8):1601–1604.

Wood, P. E., M. Milligan, D. Christ, and D. Liff (1978). Group counseling for cancer patients in a community hospital. *Psychosomatics* 19(9):555–561.

Woods, N. F., and J. A. Earp (1978). Women with cured breast cancer: a study of mastectomy patients in North Carolina. *Nursing Research* 27(5):279–285.

Wortman, C. and C. Dunkel-Schetter (1979). Interpersonal Relationships and Cancer: Wortman, C., and C. Dunkel–Schetter (1987). *Conceptual and methodological issues in the study of social support.* Hillsdale, N.J.: Erlbaum.

A Theoretical Analysis. *Journal of Social Issues* 35(1):120–155.

Wyszynski, A. A. (1990). Managing noncompliance in the "difficult" medical patient: the contributions of insight. A case report. *Psychother Psychosom* 54(4):181–186.

Yalom, I. (1995). *The Theory and Practice of Group Psychotherapy,* 4th ed. New York: Basic Books.

Yalom, I. (1980). *Existential Psychotherapy.* New York: Basic Books.

Yalom, I. D., and C. Greaves (1977). Group therapy with the terminally ill. *American Journal of Psychiatry* 134(4):396–400.

Yehuda, R., A. Elkin, K. Binder-Brynes, B. Kahana, S. M. Southwick, J. Schmeidler, and E. L. Giller, Jr. (1996). Dissociation in aging Holocaust survivors. *American Journal of Psychiatry* 153(7):935–940.

Yalom, V., and I. Yalom (1990). Brief interactive group psychotherapy. *Psychiatric Annals* 20:362–367.

Index

297